Charlotte Logan is a mother of three children, living in Lisbon, Portugal. She is the founder of @Motherspath on social media, a community where she shares her tools and wisdom gained through her life experiences and lessons. She also created a podcast Charlotte Logan well-being, where all women can recognize themselves and discover how they can be authentically happy. Charlotte was born and raised in the UK in Epsom and Brighton by a French mother and English father. She was raised vegetarian in a philosophical and spiritual Indian environment.

At the age of ten, after her parents' divorce, she moved to France with her mother and sister. Charlotte has explored and practiced many types of yoga during the past 18 years such as Bikram, Hatha, prenatal/postnatal, Iyengar, and now flow. Charlotte experienced both opposites of motherhood, painful miscarriages, and amazing natural births. She discovered through these experiences that the power wasn't out there but within us.

I dedicate this book to all the women and mothers out there. May you find support and trust within yourself to overcome any challenges that may come your way.

You are beautiful and you are whole. Never doubt your worth nor your love.

Charlotte Logan

# THE PATH TO DELIVERANCE

A Guide Through Childbirth and
Motherhood, Taking You on
the Path of Self-Love
and Acceptance

AUSTIN MACAULEY PUBLISHERS™

LONDON • CAMBRIDGE • NEW YORK • SHARJAH

A CIP catalogue record for this title is available from the British Library.

ISBN 9781035837397 (Paperback)
ISBN 9781035837403 (ePub e-book)

www.austinmacauley.com

First Published 2024
Austin Macauley Publishers Ltd®
1 Canada Square
Canary Wharf
London
E14 5AA

I am forever grateful for Bob Proctor's teachings who was a modern spiritual teacher in disguise. He helped me make the shift to living a better life and believing in big goals. I wouldn't have written this book without him. I profoundly thank Deepak Chopra for his spiritual teachings and wisdom. I continue my journey to growth everyday with his speeches. His book Creating Affluence is my bible and it followed me every day while writing my book. I thank Rebecca Campbell for putting words to my intuitions, for confirming what I had discovered within me, and giving me the strength to speak my voice.

I would like to thank all the people who have consciously and unconsciously helped me on my journey to motherhood but also to becoming a better version of myself. I am very grateful for my prenatal/postnatal yoga teacher Sophie Colombié for allowing me to shift my perception of pregnancy and childbirth. I wish to thank Anna Roy, my first midwife, who has been of great support and who helped me in ways she couldn't imagine. I am grateful for my parents for raising me in a beautiful and loving spiritual environment at a young age. I am grateful for my loving sister Megan who is always there for me. I thank my step-mother Ingrid who has always sent me hints and guided me to the path I was meant to take. I thank Emilia for taking my hand and showing me the path to healing and magic. I am very grateful to Rubin Museum of art who helped me reconnect to my spirituality when I needed it the most. I thank Tara Brach for her podcast meditations and talks which help me immensely on my spiritual path. I thank Eckhart Tolle for his talks and for putting such simple and beautiful words to some very complicated topics and truths. I thank Anne-Claire for supporting me when I needed it. I thank Marie-Aude and Sabrina for their love and sisterhood. I thank my husband Alex for always believing in me and finding the right words to help me continue no matter what. I am extremely lucky to have such love from him and my children. I am very grateful to all team members at Austin Macauley for seeing the potential in me and making this book come to life.

# Table of Contents

*When I managed to give birth all by own without an epidural for my second child, it struck me, I had just discovered something major! I had just experienced a superpower. I was a new version of myself, just as if I had awakened from a long sleep, I had awakened from ignorance. I felt the urge to share my experience on how to live pregnancy and childbirth in the present moment with mindfulness.*

*In this book, all the tools will help you take care of yourself, create a powerful bond with your baby and lead you on the path to deliverance.*

My goal is to help mothers go through the beautiful storms of motherhood with strength and harmony. But also help learn different ways of birthing and existing as a mother. Whether they went through miscarriages, whether they are a mum to be or already a mum, becoming a mother is life changing from deep within.

Rather than living motherhood block by block, we can move through it. Life is movement not a box or brick staircase.

I started my path in motherhood, lost, lonely, and I can say with an underlying trauma. Ever since, I have been wanting to grow and understand as much as possible about pregnancy, birth, and the following months with a newborn baby. We can learn to free ourselves from misbeliefs, limitations, anxiety, and fear. The environment in which we give birth, our attitude has such a big impact on ourselves but also on the future of our children.

In this book, I will talk about my journey as a mum and provide practical and nurturing tools for both type of pregnancies whether it stopped too soon, arrived to the term, and until the six months of age of your newborn child. I also go in deeper with a universal, positive, and loving approach in order to understand the larger picture of the 'self' in motherhood and set the right habits in your life.

We will see together how we can take 'care' of ourselves, see ourselves as we should, with a loving and compassionate eye. Consequently, our children will benefit from it and grow with the right seeds.

If we all take part in changing the way we treat ourselves and others, change is inevitable; change starts with the individual.

Our children are the change the world needs in the near future. A natural cycle of change and adaptation will naturally follow, thus allowing our children to get the best start in life.

This isn't just a pregnancy book, it's a book about the beautiful journey all mothers go through, a transformative life experience that comes in polar opposites. With some nurturing tools, self-love, compassion, and practical tips the journey can be lived in harmony and become 'the path to deliverance'.

# Introduction

My name is Charlotte Logan; in this book I am going to talk about my journey as a mum of three children, how I struggled, how I sometimes felt I was failing (there is actually no such thing as failure) but also how wonderful and magical motherhood is when you acknowledge your powers. I will talk a bit of myself and my experiences and discuss some fundamental topics that can help you have a clear vision of motherhood.

Motherhood in a profound way, in a conscious way, in a caring way for you, for your baby and ultimately for your environment.

I will also provide practical and nurturing tools you can use in your everyday life. The tools are easy to use and to include in your daily routine. You won't feel you are making a huge effort or feel it is unrealistic to implement in your busy mummy life.

I was born and lived in Epson Sussex, in England, until I was about six years old. My parents and I then moved to Brighton where my sister was born. I couldn't wait to become a big sister and welcome a baby in our family. I had a very happy and easy childhood.

I was raised vegetarian by my parents who had made the choice of living more in harmony with this earth. Before I was born, they had travelled to India and learnt to meditate. I was raised in a loving spiritual environment where we would regularly attend meditations, philosophical and spiritual talks.

I am grateful for being directly bathed in this larger consciousness at such a young age. It helped me ask myself the right questions all along my life. My father worked hard to become a homeopath, which was quite innovative at the time, and he dedicated himself to healing and helped many people for many years.

At nine years old, we moved to France with our mum next to Paris. At twenty-three, I moved to Paris where several years later I met my husband. We had three beautiful children together until we moved to Lisbon, Portugal in 2019 where we still live today.

Here in Portugal, right next to the ocean, is where I felt the need and desire to finish my inner work and start writing this book. My path isn't finished, as we never stop evolving and growing, especially when we embrace our spirituality and who we truly are. I have always known I had a specific mission (we all do) and it took me a long time to discover what this mission was.

If you are here with me now, it means you have the will, the desire to understand this life changing experience of becoming a mum and to be in harmony with it. I will talk about the notion of harmony as we all have a false idea of it. Or maybe you are here because you are afraid of the unknown of this life-changing experience of becoming a mother.

YOU are here now, and we will bring change together in your habits allowing you to give birth fully in connection with yourself and live your life as a parent more mindfully and with less fear.

In this book, nothing is about being perfect, it's about being your unique self. Self-development is a journey and as mothers we embody self-development! We are constantly questioning, learning, and evolving. We acquire knowledge that brings us awareness that ultimately brings us confidence and trust in our own capabilities.

I will do my very best to support you cultivate self-love. Trust yourself because there is no such thing as right or wrong as a mother. You are here now, now is all there is, and you are enough.

# Chapter One
# Journey to Motherhood

## Losing Your Baby

My journey in motherhood started by losing my first baby. I had always wanted children since I was a little girl and never would I have thought to live such an experience. I suppose for two reasons, one because I thought tragic things only happened to other people, and two, it is sadly a very taboo subject.

Luckily, it is slowly starting to come into the light. This subject is very difficult to talk about, yet it is very common in a woman's life when she desires to have children. I actually went through two miscarriages, or may I say I lost two babies. 'Miscarriage' is a term more and more people do not like to use.

I handled the loss differently as they were two very different experiences at two very different moments of my life, as a woman and a mother. I must confess, that the pain and suffering does depend on the gravity of the experience, how advanced we are in our pregnancy, the way we perceive the situation and how we handle the grieving process. It is important to deal with it, recognise it in order to free ourselves from the secret little dark box we hold deep inside our heart.

This little box should not exist, nor should it stay hidden within, it creates a lot of damage that we can avoid. We must acknowledge the experience and the emotions that come with it. I will share further on, some powerful tools that can help you do this.

My first miscarriage was with a little baby that was not planned. One could think, "oh it's less hard then," well it wasn't. I actually deeply desired this baby, even though the circumstances in my life were not ideal. I have always wanted to be a mum as far I can recall.

So, I lost this little human being at fourteen weeks and a half of pregnancy, two weeks after the first ultrasound. The first ultrasound in my life as a mother was the most magical experience I had yet lived. I saw a very happy and healthy baby jumping up and down in my tummy. I can remember the doctor saying how energic this little baby was.

However, after 2 days of cramping and not listening to the little voice inside saying: "Charlotte, this is not normal, do something," I started to bleed in the middle of the night.

At the hospital, when I was told the heart had stopped beating, my world collapsed. As we all do, as a survival reflex in dramatic situations, was to think that this could not be happening to me, that they must check twice or do something about it. But I quickly realised it was the reality and that measures had to be taken rapidly.

The doctors doing their job, first suggested to wait and see if I could give birth naturally. The wait was horrible and too long. I was alone in this depressing room with no explanation nor support and I was waiting to see if I could give birth to my dead baby.

After a very long while, a doctor barged in the room saying I had an infection, and that we had to operate urgently. I had to have a curettage done under general anaesthesia.

I waited in this corridor, lying down on a stretcher looking at the ceiling alone with my thoughts, as if I was waiting for death. In fact, I had just experienced death within me and whether it happens fourteen weeks pregnant or thirty-four weeks, the scares (wounds) never really disappear.

I learnt several weeks later that my baby was a little boy. The doctor who had operated me inadvertently told me it was a boy during a check-up appointment. The lack of tact or thought reopened this deep, unhealed wound. I had always wanted a little boy.

My second loss was eight years later; we wanted a third child with my husband. We already had two beautiful children so when my pregnancy test was positive, I wasn't worried nor expecting to live another difficult experience.

I was six weeks pregnant when I was told the heart wasn't beating and probably never did. The experience was less tragic, but I still had to process that it was happening to me again and that I now had to go through the experience of expulsing the embryo. I can remember how long the wait felt from the moment the doctors suspected the heart would never beat and the moment I would have to go through an early abortion. I can clearly remember spending a whole week-end in London with my sister with this embryo inside of me, feeling pregnant without any symptoms (the symptoms had faded away), wondering whether this baby was going to live and how I should feel. The ambivalence of my emotions and the hope I still held in my heart only added to the discomfort of a body already preparing for a baby. When I got back to Paris the ultrasound confirmed what I was dreading and what I already suspected deep inside. The hospital where I was meant to give birth gave me the abortion pills.

I had to take them at home, alone. They warned me it could take several days and that it usually was very painful. I was apprehensive and scared, luckily it went smoothly, and I didn't suffer that much. Having said this, physically it went well but it took three to four days of bleeding, cramping to finally expulsing the embryo in the toilet. I wasn't prepared for the wound it creates inside and the trauma it silently leaves behind.

My journey after these two miscarriage experiences is not an example. The fact is, I didn't handle it well. I didn't talk about it, I just hid the pain deep down to forget about it as fast as possible and pretend it never happened. This does not work; it just builds-up inside and makes a lot of damage.

It took me ten years to understand I hadn't healed, I was suffering every single day. It took me courage and the help of guides to take care of it.

## Tips and Tools for the Mind and Soul

### The notion of separateness

When I think of my first pregnancy, when I was carrying life inside me for the first time, the general sensation and feeling was separateness. Maybe the fact that the circumstances around this pregnancy weren't very positive; nevertheless, I was living the experience in a separate way. As if, as long as we can't see or physically touch something it doesn't really exist.

We talk about pregnancy more as a physical state, if I exaggerate a bit, even as if we were sick. We know in our mind and heart that we are carrying life, but in a way, it feels unreal and distant, this is the notion of separateness. There is a 'you' and there is a 'me'; it's not surprising as we live in a world of separateness and ego.

I now realise that when I lost this little baby, I was more 'next' to this baby not 'with'. When we, women, are pregnant, we are a 'we', we are a 'with', a oneness. And whether we lose our baby too soon or whether we give birth, the notion of oneness and togetherness is very important.

## Do not let this become a taboo subject

The first and most primordial advice I can give you is to seek for help. It can be a member of your family, your husband or a psychiatrist but talk about it. What did you feel? How do you feel now? My family and husband were there for me, but they couldn't fill the emptiness I felt inside.

Very rapidly everyone around us, to protect us, act as if this baby or pregnancy never existed. Just as if this life we carried in our womb, disappears with time, until the point where this life never really existed. You don't or can't talk about it and when you bring it up people get uncomfortable and turn their heads away.

Again, your baby went from the tangible to the intangible but he or she existed, and you are free to acknowledge her or him and talk about it as long as you need to.

I chose to see a Jungian psychologist. I was in depression, I had panic attacks and my body was sending me all sorts of signals that I had to take care of myself. I saw my therapist for about five years and it saved me on many levels. It helped me with most of the grieving process and it gave me the trust in myself again.

*Jungian psychology: Carl Gustav Jung was a Swiss psychiatrist most known for his theories of personal and collective unconscious and extraversion and introversion. He believed that religious expression was manifested from the psyche's yearning for a balanced state of consciousness and unconsciousness simultaneously.*

*Dreams are very important in Jungian psychology, it is a good way to understand the emotions and habitual behaviour patterns we may have. Carl Jung's theory is the collective unconscious. He believed that human beings are connected to each other and their ancestors through a shared set of experiences. We use this collective consciousness to give meaning to the world.*

### Mourning prayer

I discovered very late, ten years later, that it was very important to mourn and consciously recognise and accept what happened. But when you lose your child before the third trimester, there is no event nor ceremony to pray and say goodbye.

I am not a Catholic, but I have a special connection to churches. So, when I was told to find a place to pray and finally close the wound in my heart and soul, I intuitively knew where I wanted to go. My husband and I went to this little church in our neighbourhood called in Portuguese 'Nossa Senhora dos Anjos', *Our Lady of the Angels*. Yes, if you pay attention to your intuition, it will often make you smile and bring you to the right places.

We could finally both grieve, we could both say: "You existed, we love you and always will, be free."

For those who have experienced the terrible loss of their baby at the end of their pregnancy term or during the first days of life at the hospital, a funeral is planned. It may be enough for some and in that case, no need to push further. However, if you feel the slight need that it wasn't quite enough, do your own mourning prayer or symbolic ritual.

### Symbolic ritual

What ritual could you think of to honour the memory of your lost child and let his/her soul be free? There are many ways to create a symbolic ritual and I encourage you to take the time to think about it and let your heart speak to you. I have a few examples, like planting a tree, or writing a letter you put in a bottle and sending it out to sea with your thoughts of love, writing a poem and reading it out loud on a full moon. Whatever vibrates within you, do it; create your own symbolic ritual.

### Spiritual approach

This child existed and will always exist for you. His or her body has left you but his or her soul, spiritual essence, will always exist and will always be there for you. Think of it as a pact you had with this soul, you already knew each other, and you were meant to live this experience together. You will find peace and you will be happy again.

I know my first son is my guardian angel, he protects me and guides me. He brings me peace and allows me to feel joy and happiness again. I know you feel guilt when you laugh or feel happy, you already feel guilty losing your child and not being able to do anything about it. But you are allowed to have joy in your life again and this is what your angel baby wants for you.

## Mindful grieving meditation

The best way to reconnect to yourself, to find that peace or most importantly start to grieve and heal, is to do short meditation exercises on a daily basis or every other day. It doesn't have to be long, twenty minutes can do the trick. It may be hard at first; strong emotions will probably surface, you will cry, you may feel deep anxiety. I know how scary this can feel but you are not alone, and you can find that comforting warmth inside you.

If it is too overwhelming, which can happen, don't push it, try another day when you are ready. You do need this time for you, and it will heal you with time, but be patient and gentle with yourself. Once you are ready and it becomes a habit, you will feel and understand all the benefits of meditating.

Find your quiet spot where you won't be disturbed. Light a candle, sit with your back straight, make sure you feel comfortable but awake. Close your eyes and listen to your breath. Sit with yourself, feel the sensations in your body. If it's too much emotionally and you feel anxious, you can keep your eyes open and concentrate on the candle flame. Focus on the sounds around you rather than on your breath.

To open the meditation, take a deep breath, fill your lungs and heart area, fill your abdomen. When you exhale, exhale with a sound or strong sigh. Let go of your thoughts and tensions. Do this three times. Now you can scan each part of your body and try to release any tension you may have in your muscles or in your sitting posture.

You can put a hand on your heart and breathe normally. You will have images and thoughts come to you constantly, it is normal; don't fix your attention on it or feel guilty. Just let the thoughts pass with kindness and focus back on your breath or sounds.

I learnt through the Rubin Museum meditation podcast with a spiritual Buddhist teacher, Lama Aria Drolma, that the colour blue in Tibetan Buddhism represents deep healing. Now, imagine a blue ball of light in front you, the colour is pure like a fresh mint sweet and you can feel it's soothing power. Listen to your breath and imagine inhaling the blue light, it goes to all parts of your body, it touches each cell.

After as many breaths as you need when you breathe out, see your sorrow and pain float away and be taken care of by this beautiful blue light, healing you, breath after breath. A thought will pop-up; it's alright, don't block it, let it pass. You can come back at any time and do this over and over again.

In your own time, come back to noticing the sensations in your body; if emotions arise, just let them be. You are safe within yourself, you are not alone. When you are ready, slowly move your fingertips and toes and open your eyes.

You can also go right to page 136 where I provide a similar but different meditation guidance, I also give some meditation podcast recommendations.

## Energetician therapist

I finished the grieving process many years later with an energetician therapist who worked with crystal and quartz stones. This technique allows energy blockages in your body to dissolve and create a harmonious balance from within. The Universe and its beings are made of energy, it needs to flow.

I had many energy blockages that needed to be treated so I could fully heal. I had several sessions and each one of them was extremely revealing and powerful. It's also a moment of deep relaxation and selfcare that is essential when you lost a baby. A session usually lasts an hour or so.

The energetician therapist will ask you some questions and then you lie down on a massage table where the treatment begins. The therapist will place stones on different parts of your body, corresponding to the different chakras. The therapist will then scan your body with his/her hands and work the energy through your body.

Ask around you if someone knows a good energetician, word of mouth is a great way. You must feel comfortable with the therapist to be able to let go and fully trust. It's just like a psychologist, you must feel at ease, and that it's the right person for you.

## Walks

Allow some time for yourself where you can go for walks in the nature, in the woods, near a river or on the beach. Focus on the beauty of what you see, listen to the sounds, be aware of the smells, become part of it. Try focusing on the present, on the now, because now is all there is. In the now, there is

YOU, connect with the elements around you. As Rumi says: "When you feel beauty, you know it as truth."

I always feel happy and grateful when I am in the nature, whether it's in a forest or on a beach. There is something very simple and pure that happens in those moments and it nourishes your heart and soul. You can also let go, fully acknowledge your mourning and your pain. Whisper like a prayer and trust that the earth and trees around you can hear you. Know that they will take care of your deep sorrows.

### Massage

Book yourself an essential oil massage to reconnect with your body to give time to heal. Your body has been through a tsunami, tension and sorrow, which is held in your tissues and muscles; you must allow the tension to melt away. Essential oils are very powerful and specific oils can be used to heal your mind and body. Find an essential oil massage therapist near you.

If you don't find anyone specialised, a gentle full body massage with natural oils is just as good. You can also have a look at page 158 where I give a list of the essential oils you can use in your bath to safely take care of yourself.

### Homeopathy

As I said, my father was a homeopath in the UK for twenty-five years. I grew-up with homeopathy and my father treated everyone at home. I am not against general medicine, and I do use both. Homeopathy is particularly efficient and interesting for emotional problems and long-term symptoms that are usually caused by unhealed emotional wounds, anxiety or stress in our daily life.

When you see a homeopath, you will talk about your physical symptoms but also your emotions. It is a good moment to open-up and share what you have locked-up inside. To help you heal your heart and soul after your traumatic experience, homeopathy can be a very good ally. Find a homeopath from word to mouth or ask for some advice around you.

## Simple yoga and stretching exercises

You can do the following four yoga exercises daily to stretch-out, relax and gently strengthen your core muscles. Your body needs to smoothly wake-up, your perineum (your pelvic floor) needs moderate re-education. No matter the number of months you were pregnant, the idea here is to reconnect, feel the sensations in your body.

Yet do this in a gentle and respectful way, not pushing your body nor limits. You can do the following exercise cycle three times.

You will need: a yoga mat, a yoga block or two, and some cushions.

## Downward facing dog pose (Adho Mukha Svanasana)

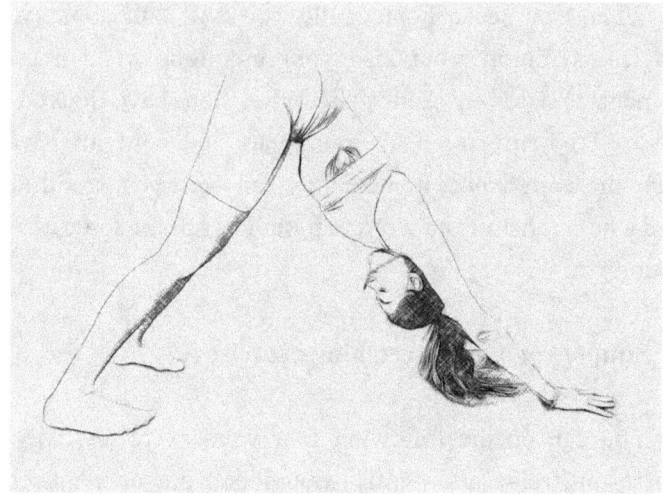

Stand-up your legs slightly larger than your hips. Bend down to form a bridge face facing down. Put your hands flat on the floor with your fingers open like a star, anchor your hands in the ground. Your heels don't have to touch the floor, if you can't it's fine, leave some space. Now push on your hands, arms straight and dynamic, as if you wanted to push the top of your bottom in the air and backwards.

Let your head be heavy and drop down, breathe. Your legs are straight and strong, your back is straight. To make sure your back is straight, pull your pelvis slightly in and your belly is pulled towards your back. There is no effort in your abdominal muscles. Stay like this for fifteen seconds, then come-up on your feet, slowly unrolling your spine, vertebrate after vertebrate, from the bottom to the top of your head.

## Perineal exhale (lying down)

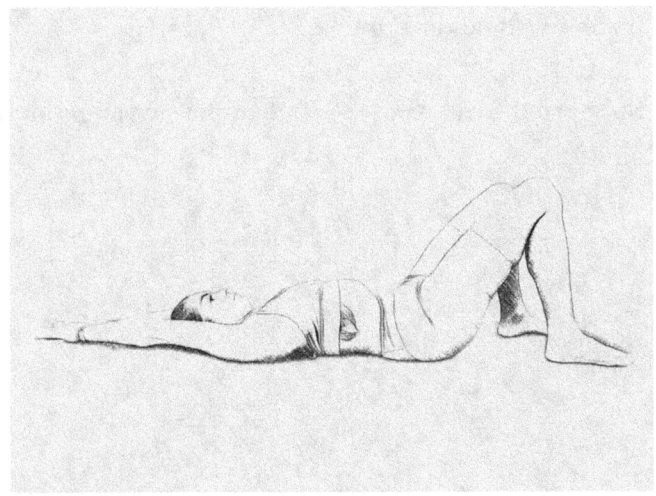

I learnt this technique in prenatal yoga classes with Sophie Colombié in Paris. This technique is magic and can be used to gently re-educate your perineum.

Lie down on your yoga or gym mat, bend your knees keeping your feet on the ground. Breathe in while bringing your hands together, hook your index fingers together. While you exhale, bring your arms above your head, arms straight and strong as if your wanted to reach the wall behind you.

Come back while inhaling and start again but this time while you exhale, bring your arms above your head, push with your feet on the floor. You will feel your back flatten and your belly sink in. This posture retroverts your pelvis and mechanically pulls-up your perineum. Your perineum needs gentle awakening and protection after what you have been through.

Stay like this for fifteen seconds, then come back while inhaling. Breathe normally. Repeat as many times as you like, minimum five times in a row.

**Supported Bridge pose (Setu bandha sarvangasana)**

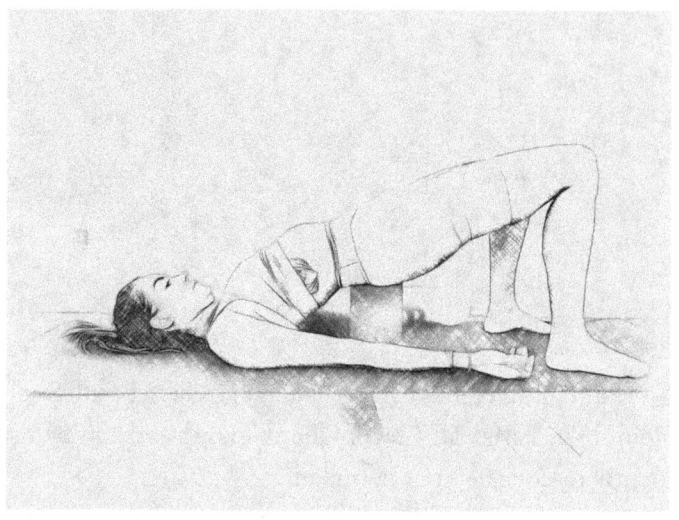

This posture is wonderful for opening the heart area and great for your shoulders and your back. You will need a yoga block.

Lie on your mat, bend your knees, take a block and place it long length standing-up under your sacrum (lower back, just above your bottom). Cross your hands and fingers together under your body, arms straight. Now push your shoulders outwards towards the ground as if you wanted both of your shoulder blades to join in your back.

Your breasts and thorax are going upwards and opening wide. Keep your chin towards your neck, touching your thorax. Make sure your knees are not leaning outwards, bring them inwards and keep them straight. Remember to breathe, stay for two to three minutes, and come back down slowly, unrolling your spine, vertebrate after vertebrate, starting from your cervical right down to your bottom/sacrum.

**Supported butterfly pose (Supta baddha konasana)**

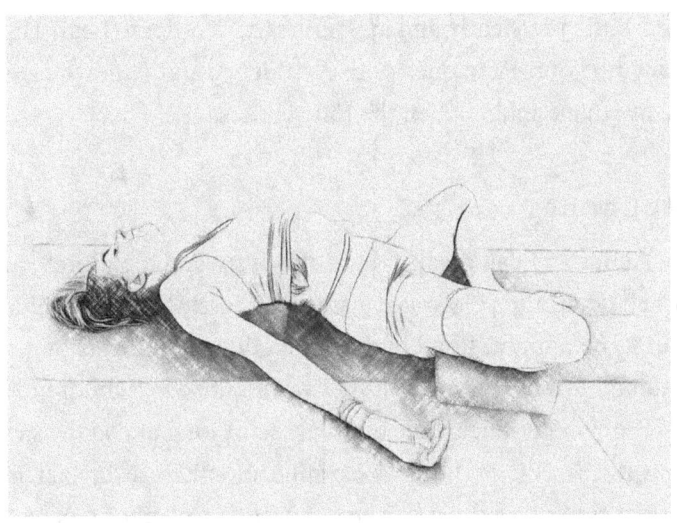

You will need one or two yoga blocks and two cushions.

Place a block on your mat where your back and shoulder blades will be. Lie down on your mat and make sure the block is flat, large side parallel to the top width of your mat. The block should be in the middle of your shoulder blades, place the block quite low so your shoulders drop backwards towards the floor. Your thorax is open, feel your heart beating and breathe.

Join your feet together and bring them towards you against your pelvis, your feet stay on the floor. Now open your knees and let them drop on each side, place a cushion under each knee to give some support to the opening and pulling of the muscles. You are opening your pelvis groins (counternutation). Spread-out your arms on each side and breathe.

Inside your body you are closing your pelvis, energetically closing the birth passage. You can visualise with your eyes closed, a canal or path closing. You are only closing for a while physically and in your heart, in order to heal. Thus, allowing yourself to open with confidence and faith when you are pregnant again, when the time comes.

## Pregnancy

As far as I can recall, I have always wanted children, and to be specific, I've always wanted three children. I couldn't wait to be a mum. I had high expectations and ideals on how I wanted to give birth and how I would raise my children.

From experience, nine months seems long and at the same time it goes by so fast. These nine months are in fact just perfect timing, and we can use this time to truly prepare for birth and for the arrival of our baby. We can use this time to learn how to connect to our body and connect with our baby. Doing so, we are preparing to experience childbirth in a more balanced and grounded way.

No matter how our childbirth experience turns out, we are present and ready. I will share my experiences and tools so you can choose what inspires you and apply it in your everyday life, during the nine following months, so you are fully prepared on THE day.

After I got married, I was desperate to get pregnant again and to feel those magical sensations within me. I couldn't wait to create and carry life inside me again. After losing a baby and going through the traumatising experience of a miscarriage, I wanted my husband to be able to take part and support me during this pregnancy. I decided to try haptonomy sessions with my gynaecologist, who was also a haptonomy practitioner.

## What Is Haptonomy?

I wanted to find a way to create a connection with my baby and for my husband to create a bond with our child too. It's also important for the partner to feel part of the pregnancy and connect in a different way. During a session, you and your partner learn 'touch and feel' techniques (that's how I call it). With your hands and energy, you delicately communicate with your baby.

You can then do it at home once a day with your partner. It becomes your special time together, where you, your partner and your baby(s) connect. The response(s) you experience with your child is beyond amazing.

Albert Goldberg, a practitioner in Paris, explains that: "Haptonomy takes prenatal life very seriously. It helps the mother to deepen the intuitive contact she has with her baby from within, to prepare for birth and to share this relationship with Dad."

While the notion of separation or 'apart' is very strong in this world, finding ways to connect and become one is primordial while being pregnant. Knowing these techniques, you will be able to talk to your baby and communicate with him or her during labour and childbirth. Your child being used to your contact and 'messages' will respond in an invisible and magical way.

## Mindful Prenatal Meditation

I approach meditation several times in this book because it's a beautiful tool that can be used in each phase or situation of motherhood. Prenatal meditation has amazing effects on your wellbeing and will be felt by your baby in utero. It is a way to start communicating and bonding with your baby before birth.

Sit in a comfortable position where you wish, either on your bed, on a cushion or on your sofa. If you sit with your legs crossed, support each knee with a cushion so there is no tension. If crossing your legs is difficult (being at the end of your pregnancy), choose the position that feels right for you. Close your eyes, or if you prefer to keep a low gaze.

Start by breathing-in deeply, filling-up your lungs and then exhaling nice and slow. Do this three times. Start to scan your body from head to toe. Start with your forehead, relax the eyebrows and the back of your eyes. Make sure your jaw is relaxed. You can bring a slight smile to the lips if you wish.

Continue to scan down your body, relax your neck, your shoulders, your higher back and your torso. If there is any tightness there, breathe in that area as if you were filling your heart and lungs with beautiful yellow light.

If any thoughts show-up, which they will, it is fine just let them pass and refocus on your breath. You can put your hands on your belly and start to feel your breathing. Try and feel your tummy expanding, both on the sides and at the front.

Breathe naturally without forcing anything. Continue to scan down your body from your lower back right down to your toes.

Take the time to do this properly, thinking and feeling in each part of your body.

Now come back to your tummy. Imagine your baby inside your tummy being attentive to what you are doing and how you are feeling. Your baby is inside you and is part of you, sharing this vibrational field. All around us there is a vibrational field we can't see, but we can feel it when we sit in meditation and focus on our breath or sounds around us.

It is the perfect opportunity to feel the oneness with your baby. Using this peaceful moment, you can then expand your body to the room, feel it. Then imagine you are expanding to the outdoors and now even further to the whole planet.

Again, don't feel guilty or block your thoughts, they are here to remind us to refocus. If you feel like it, you can use a simple haptonomy exercise to communicate with your child. Place both hands on each side of your belly. With your right hand, palm flat on your tummy, light as a feather, press very gently towards your tummy counting to five and then release the action very slowly, counting to five.

Repeat this movement three to four times. It's a bit as if you were imitating the flow of the ocean by creating a soft wave. You can do the same on the other side of your tummy with your left hand. Very often you will notice your baby responding to your touch by coming against your hand and even pushing energetically against your tummy. Your baby is communicating and answering to your touch.

You can do this a few times. Don't insist if your baby is not responding. He/she could be sleeping or is simply not in the mood to respond.

You may stroke your belly to say thank you and refocus on your breath. When you are ready, you can open your eyes and slowly start moving your body.

## Prenatal Loving Kindness Meditation

Loving kindness is a different type of meditation often used in mindful meditation. The first steps are the same as mindful meditation but then we are guided to feel, see and send loving kindness to ourselves first, then to all human beings and the earth.

Sit in a comfortable position where you wish, either on your bed, on a cushion or on your sofa. If you sit with your legs crossed, support each knee with a cushion. If crossing your legs is difficult being at the end of your pregnancy, choose the position that feels right for you.

Close your eyes or keep a low gaze. Start to scan through your body, starting from the top of your head. Relax the muscles in your forehead, scan down to your eyes and notice how much tension there is there. Go down to your lips, mouth, and jaw, gently relax. You can open your mouth wide, three to four times to help you release the tension in the micro muscles. Scan down your neck to your shoulders.

I know I hold a lot of tension there. Even though, you are relaxed, notice how you can let go a little more in this area. Breathe in three deep breaths, counting to five on the inhale and five on the exhale. Now scan down to your torso and heart, focus on your breathing in this area and the sensation in your chest.

Imagine with your breath that you are creating space as if your chest was round and light like a balloon. Now scan down your entire back focusing on your spine and try to let go and breathe in the spots where you have tension or pain.

Focus on your tummy, you can put your hands on your belly if you wish. It's harder when you are pregnant because your tummy won't sink in when you let go of the tightness but try and visualise and feel your abdominal muscles soften and your organs rest. Continue to browse down to your lower back.

When we are pregnant, the lower back is a very sensitive and fragile spot. Try and see how you can let go with your breath by breathing in deep and slow. While you exhale, imagine your hips and lower back widen and open to the space around you, your bottom sinking in the ground beneath you. Let go of your thighs, knees, down to your feet right to the tip of your toes.

Now concentrate on your breath, you can focus on your abdomen, chest, or nostrils. If focusing on the breathing is uncomfortable, focus on the noises around you, in the room and in the distance.

Now, imagine a big ball of golden white light in front of you. This light is pure love, compassion, and kindness. To help you feel while visualising, think of someone you love with all your heart and who makes you smile. Now try and stay in that feeling and imagine this beautiful white light shine towards you with all this love and compassion.

It radiates through your entire body and fills your heart up. Now give yourself this love and loving kindness, feel it for your being. Now repeat this phrase ten to fifteen times: 'May I be happy, may I be safe, may I be strong'. It is very important you start sending love to yourself first before directing it to someone else.

After you repeated this to yourself, think of someone you would like to send this love to. To help you, you can visualise sending this pure white light.

Then, imagine sending it to one or several people who are troubling you. If you find it hard, you don't need to stay there long. Go back to feeling this genuine loving kindness for yourself, for a loved one and repeat: "May we be happy, may we be safe, may we be strong." Now send it to the entire planet and all its beings. Visualise the light bathing and surrounding the entire earth.

For a few minutes, stay there and then gently come back to the sensations in your body, and the sounds around you. Before opening your eyes, slowly start moving your fingers, hands and your feet. Open your eyes and enjoy this feeling as long as you wish or can.

## Pro-Social States of Mind

I didn't really know what pro-social states of mind meant when I heard about it in Dan Harris' documentary, *The Dalai Lama's guide to happiness.* He and Richard Davidson, the neuroscientist, explain that everything we do, we do it for others too. What does that mean?

They give the following examples: when we work, we make money for ourselves but also for our family, to take care of others. Or, when we eat to be strong, we also eat to be able to be of service to others. We don't naturally think of it this way, but it is so true. Everything we do, is for others too. If we remind ourselves to be more altruist throughout the day, it makes us happier.

Giving and sharing with others makes us happier, so every insignificant action we take during the day, is for ourselves but very often it's for others too. We are not meant to be alone nor feel separate. We are social animals, who need each other to evolve and thrive. We unconsciously do all these things but once we are aware of this, we can consciously put the intention in our daily life.

Before any daily activity, you can dedicate it to yourself but also to others. We don't need to be a spiritual person or a wise monk to be more present with ourselves and with others. These attributes are also trainable through meditation. With the aid of meditation, we can change. These are wonderful exercises you can do pregnant because your child will directly benefit from it.

There is no doubt, that when you express these intentions and develop a deeper sense of altruism, that your child inherits the features.

Having said this, it is also important to know that yes, we also feel negative emotions. You may ask yourself, what happens if my baby feels them too? I know I felt stressed and guilty when I didn't feel happy nor compassionate. When we hear that our baby can feel our emotions or intentions, it can create a lot of anxiety.

But we don't live in a fairy tale where everything is pink, sparkly and happy every day. There are days or periods where we may feel anxious, sad, or angry. We feel a huge range of emotions because we are human. It is natural and it is not a bad thing, every emotion has an opposite. We must accept it, feel OK with our emotion, let it exist and let it pass.

When you feel ready, work towards the opposite emotion. So, for example if you feel anxious, the opposite emotion is serenity. Try and work towards this feeling, even if it's just a little bit.

You must also know that positive emotions are far stronger and powerful than negative emotions. So, if you feel happy, or love even for a few hours, you are charging up your internal battery and sweeping away all the other less positive feelings. Knowing you can train to feel more balanced within with meditation and pro-social states of mind, this worry and anxiety of your baby feeling your emotions, will simply disappear.


## Jungian Therapist

Whether your pregnancy is physically going smoothly, it can sometimes bring up anxiety or strong emotions. Or maybe you are going through some complications. In this case, sometimes mediation or self-love is just not enough, there are deeper emotions or traumas that need to be seen for more clarity and it is alright to ask for the help.

I was very busy with my property management company in Paris when I was pregnant with my son. I worked long hours and carried heavy things around in the day-to-day maintenance and logistic of my business. I wasn't too concerned whether I was doing too much or not, I always thought I was tough and that I didn't need to take time for myself nor listen to my needs.

I was anxious and I feared another miscarriage, and yet being a young entrepreneur, I thought I could handle it all.

I remember distinctly that Christmas morning, when I discovered slight bleeding. I was in panic and this time with my husband, we rushed to the hospital where I was registered to give birth. The monitoring showed contractions even though the bleeding had stopped. They kept me in the hospital for five days and gave me a treatment for high blood pressure; this is the treatment hospitals prescribe to stop the contractions.

The major issue was to slow down the contractions, they didn't want my cervix to shorten and eventually open. I was hardly six months pregnant, so the doctor didn't want to take any unnecessary risk and he decided I should stop all physical activity including work.

At this point, I was so frightened, anxiety was showing-up again, old emotions from my miscarriage were coming-up to the surface, and all I could feel was fear down to my soul. Luckily, my Jungian therapist was there to help me; she guided me to find the trust and confidence I had in me.

If you have a risky pregnancy, if you have old traumas showing-up, or anxiety of the future, it is very important to seek for help and not stay alone. If you don't take care of things when you feel them, sure enough your body will send you the signs later on. Talking to or being heard by a therapist can free you from future repressed emotions and fear.

A therapist is someone neutral and who genuinely is there to help you nurture your inner nature. I prefer Jungian therapists, who work by listening to the signs your body is sending you and by analysing your dreams (the subconscious). I have known my Jungian therapist for thirteen years now. You must feel comfortable with your therapist, listen to your intuition or your guts.

If something is off with the first person you see, just look for someone else. There are enough good therapists out there adapted for each and one of us.

To come back to my pregnancy, the last trimester was long, actually very long, but at least I had time for me, time to rest, time to prepare my nest for the long-desired child. The more advanced I was in my pregnancy and the more relaxed I became.

## Nesting

It is actually something we naturally do in the last trimester of pregnancy. Some say it is usually around the 38th week of pregnancy because your body is preparing for childbirth. I felt it much earlier than that.

For my third pregnancy, I started reorganising my kids' bedrooms four months before childbirth. I remember I found an old desk in the dumpster of our building, and I just loved it! I was five months pregnant when I started to sand it down and paint it to give it an Art Deco style, now it makes a great desk for my son.

So nesting is this urge to reorganise the house, to prepare the nursery, make sure the list of things we will need for baby is complete. In fact, just like animals, it's an instinct, it's in our genes. Welcoming a baby, is a very powerful and intimate moment in one's life, so it is important to make it comfortable, cosy and to your image.

Ultimately, creating a nurturing and comfortable home for you and your baby is a way of taking care of yourself. The inside of your home is just like the inside of your heart, it's your well-being. In this life changing experience of having a baby, your well-being is precious, and needs to be taken care of.

Now just remember to take it easy, and save some time to rest and listen to your body. That's why starting early gives you time to do it with no rush. Don't take any unnecessary risks and let your husband participate and do the heavy lifting or building. Dads need to feel useful and prepare for the arrival of their baby too.

## What If I'm Not Nesting?

You may not feel this at all and it's fine. You may be ready without knowing or you have a natural 'go with the flow', which is beautiful. As long as you feel happy and that your home is welcoming and nurturing for you and your baby.

If it's not, ask for help around you. Your husband can do much more than us women allow our men to do. Ask a member of your family or a close friend to create a cosy and comfortable atmosphere to your living room, bedroom and/or your nursery. Just a good clean, reorganisation and sorting out can do the trick. I feel great when I sort out my house and give things away or sell what can be sold.

Also, it doesn't need to cost much. I know society and social media makes us think that we must have the best things and spend lots of money. Well, if you can't (and even if you could), I don't recommend to. You can buy second-hand furniture, clothes, and equipment. And if you want, buy some brand new, because it's good to find the balance in everything we do.

You can buy some reasonable new decoration items just for that satisfaction and contentment feeling. Just make your home or some of the rooms a clean slate, it doesn't have to be the whole house.

## Midwife/Prenatal Accompaniment

During this third trimester, a midwife was visiting me at home twice a week to make sure my cervix was doing well, and that my baby was comfortable and healthy. I had the best midwife in Paris, Anna Roy! She helped me trust myself that I could give birth the way I wanted to, which was the most naturally and physiologically possible.

I didn't want an epidural and I wanted to be able to walk around the birth room and find the position that suited me and my baby. I also wanted to give birth in the water, if my labour conditions allowed it. I must mention that I chose one of the most open-minded maternity hospitals in Paris, 'Les Bluets'.

They are one of the best in terms of natural birth methods and a less medicalized environment and yet separated by a corridor with a larger hospital that has all the medical equipment required if a vital emergency arises. Wanting to be more in touch with your body and baby doesn't mean you reject medical assistance and the staff.

I have always been very grateful for their work and knowledge. We need them, and I truly thank them. It's just a matter of giving one's choice, being open, more flexible to the mother's desire and creating a warmer and more welcoming environment.

Anna Roy was also there to listen to me and give me all sorts of advice but also a lot of comfort. We can be very emotional and sensitive especially at the end of our pregnancy and we need the compassion and support.

I sometimes felt very lonely and having a midwife or a prenatal accompaniment is very important for the construction of a happy and confident mummy.

*Anna Roy is a midwife who works in the 4th arrondissement of Paris and at the time worked at the 'Bluets' maternity hospital where I gave birth. She has come a long way since she now does a chronicle in a French TV show 'La Maison des Maternelles' about maternity and children.*

*Anna has her own Podcast 'Sage-Meuf' on a French radio, Europe 1. She is also an author of numerous books on pregnancy, baby care and storytelling of her experiences in her profession as a midwife.*

*She is also raising her voice to improve the conditions of her profession as a midwife and make sure quality accompaniment can be assured to mothers in labour and allow birth in a harmonious environment. Anna Roy is an optimist activist who is asking for more staff (1 midwife = 1 woman) so there is less damage and mistakes made to the families, to create and allow more private and intimate birth settings and stop gynaecological and obstetrical violences.*

Anna believes things can change fast and I strongly support her voice because if mothers can give birth in caring and trusting ways, then the children we bring into this world will be born with the fundamental values one needs in life.

As Deepak Chopra says in his book, *Creating Affluence:* "Without values, there is confusion and chaos. (...) Health disintegrates, poverty attains dominance over affluence, societies and civilisations crumble."

I have not had the experience of a doula or prenatal accompaniment, but I think it can really help feeling listened to, having someone who can guide you through your pregnancy and childbirth, and this depending on your personal needs. It's like having a 'big sister' available just for you all along the way, someone who has the experience and the right theoretical tools. It's also someone who can bring you a spiritual and more connected approach to childbirth.

Overall, it's making sure you are not alone. We can feel very lonely and vulnerable when we are pregnant, no matter how many children you have. It is not a moment of separateness but one of 'oneness'. One with your child, one with someone there for you, who's unique interest is your well-being as well as your baby's.

*My friend, Justine, finished her course in prenatal accompaniment in Paris. She is a mum of three and is based in Lisbon, Portugal.*

# Children

*Children when they are born are pure,*
*they are an expression of love, they are souls.*
*They are the proof of the magic of life,*
*the proof of the existence of the divine.*
*We must protect the future love of this planet.*

*Charlotte Logan*

For my second pregnancy, my first daughter, I was actively working again. I was more confident in my capabilities, and I was also more in tune with what I could do. It was the beginning of a fragile balance between working, being active and taking time for me.

Of course, it is not easy when you already have a young child (my son was three years old at the time). I had help from my husband and I reorganised my time as much as I could.

Having said this, I wasn't taking days off, but I was introducing small new habits in my life, listening to my needs. For example, I am a coffee lover, and I can remember I would drop-off my son at preschool and stop at the coffee roaster shop next door. This was a real treat for me before starting my busy day.

I would choose my coffee blend, and take fifteen minutes just for me, smell the roasted coffee beans in the air, take time to breath and watch people rush to work through the small coffee window.

Another thing that makes me happy is having my warm baths. I took them less hot than I usually would and I would put some essential oils (see page 147 for use recommendations) or I would treat myself with some fun and colourful 'Lush' foam bars.

Time won't be given to you, but you can take the time. Fifteen minutes won't ruin your workday, but it will do you and your baby a lot of good.

## Yoga

I can't remember how I got to start **prenatal yoga classes** and how I found Sophie Colombié, but she is just amazing! She literally switched the perception I had of my own body and the power of women during childbirth.

*Sophie Colombié graduated from the Sivananda school, trained in India and Europe. She is specialised in the teaching of yoga for pregnant women.*

*Coming from contemporary dance, Sophie is passionate about vitality, well-being, movement, and the potential for bodily, mental, and spiritual development of individuals. The possibility of feeling, of knowing, of freeing and opening the body enthuses and animates her.*

I would go to her classes at least once a week and then twice a week at the end of my pregnancy. Very quickly, I realised she would mention during the classes something I was aware of, but I had completely underestimated the importance of: the perineum.

Sophie would teach us breathing techniques inspired by Bernadette de Gasquet's work that associated the perineum and the opening of the pelvis called: perineum exhale.

Basically, Sophie told us there were just a few yoga/breathing postures we needed to master in order to give birth the most naturally and smoothly possible. It's all about listening to your body and deeply accompanying the natural work.

*Bernadette de Gasquet is a French doctor and yoga teacher. She is the pioneer in pre-natal yoga classes and how to use and protect the perineum. In the 2000s, she developed maternal-foetal biomechanics according to birthing positions. She would work closely with midwives in the hospitals sharing her knowledge of yoga, to help women give birth the most physiologically possible.*

*Maternities wanted to train quickly in these new practices (80% of maternities trained in France), as well as many schools and many liberal midwives. She created the 'De Gasquet Institute', where she shares her precious work and offers classes for individuals and training for professionals. She has written many books and has extended her work to the general well-being of the body and mind.*

The coincidence was, that Bernadette de Gasquet was giving consultations in perinatology at 'Les Bluets' maternity hospital, where all three of my children were born. I chose this hospital because it was famous in Paris for its open-mindedness in childbirth positions, labour motion flexibility, and was pro-breastfeeding.

It was a very 'avant-garde' maternity hospital where there were very few spaces and a long waiting list. I was very lucky to have a space for each of my children.

I knew about the perineum, having done re-education sessions for the perineum after the birth of my first child. However, I had no idea how important it was to know how to use it during labour and how to protect it after birth. Luckily, in France, the perineum re-education is taken very seriously, and I was trained efficiently by my yoga teacher, Sophie.

Don't worry, I will get to it and I will share my tips and tools with you the most clearly as possible, so you can learn how to use these breathing and anatomy postures at home. I will talk about it in depth in the following chapter 'Labour and childbirth'. I also encourage you to do some research and see if you have a prenatal yoga teacher familiar with the 'perineum exhale' or the 'Bernadette de Gasquet' approach in your area.

For my third pregnancy, I had stopped working to raise my two children. With experience and being more mature in age, I felt much more confident and relaxed. This was also what I had always dreamed of, this was my dream come true, being a mother of three. However, pregnancies being like children, the ride can be very different from one pregnancy to the other.

The three first months were quite typical with the heavy nausea and feeling completely drained and exhausted. But I was a happy 'home mum'.

It was summer and we were in our summer house when I lost a clot of blood in the shower. Being three months pregnant, I obviously thought I was losing my baby again. I can remember telling myself: "No, Charlotte, this can NOT be happening again." The emergency doctors on the phone said if I had no cramping nor pain, I should lie down and just wait before rushing to the hospital to see how things evolve.

Not wanting to take the slightest risk after my miscarriages and my tricky pregnancy with my eldest, my husband drove me to the hospital.

After a long wait and a lot of worrying, the ultrasound confirmed that all was fine. I later discovered during my first official ultrasound that the bleeding and clot of blood was due to the placenta being very low and partially covering my cervix. It's called 'placenta praevia' and it can also imply having a caesarean, which I really wanted to avoid.

But if it was the safest for my baby and me, so be it. Apparently, this physical particularity often happens when you have had many pregnancies and when you get older. I was also warned that it could cause bleeding during the pregnancy but also during childbirth.

Ultimately, my pregnancy went smoothly. I had some heart issues during the last trimester that felt quite worrying. But after some tests, the cardiologist told me that it was nothing alarming and that my body was simply telling me that it was getting tired. Tachycardia is actually quite common during the last months of pregnancy but if it gets very uncomfortable and strong, it must be followed by a specialist.

Your heart is basically pumping far more blood than usual and is working with double effort to provide for your baby.

My ultrasound practitioner was very professional and precocious, but she was far from reassuring and rather alarming after each consultation. My 'Praevia' situation wasn't that bad, but she did make it a big deal and it created unnecessary stress for me and my baby. I tried to stay confident and calm but it did create quite a lot of anxiety within me.

I had all these questions in my head: "Will I have a caesarean? Will I dangerously bleed if I give birth naturally? Will I arrive in time at the hospital? And what if there are massive traffic jams when I go into labour?" etc. Luckily, I was taking my prenatal yoga classes with Sophie again which helped me trust my body and my baby.

Sophie saved me with her graceful confidence that with the postures she was showing us during the classes, and rehearsing the 'perineum exhale' exercise at home, my placenta would move upwards and leave enough space for a natural birth.

Once more, I discovered that my body and mind were so powerful, and that with the right exercises and the right mindset, you can do miracles. You just need to work with your body and let it flow, connect to a deeper knowing. I will always be amazed how magical and powerful it is to connect mind, body, and soul.

## Taking Naps

For all my pregnancies, I felt exhausted during the first three months and taking naps when I could or going to bed at eight in the evening was my favourite thing. Usually during the second trimester, we feel a boost of energy and get along just fine with our life just as it was before. In the third trimester, we start to feel heaving, tired, and out of breath.

For my fourth pregnancy (third baby), I remember to love taking naps again in the afternoon before I picked-up my other two children from school. I would lie on my bed under a comfy and soft cover and set my alarm for four pm. The school was five minutes away, so I made the most of it!

Strangely enough, I didn't feel ashamed nor guilty to take naps when I was pregnant, because it was for my baby first and because I listened to myself much more. That is when I realised that when I am not pregnant, I don't listen to my needs as much nor does it feel legitimate do so. My thinking mode just tells me that I have no time and that it's ridiculous to take naps for no reason. This is a lack of self-care and self-love.

May your pregnancy give you permission to be gentle with yourself and loving. To help you develop the habit of taking care of yourself, for you but also for others, there's the pro-social state of mind again. Continue to train yourself to these new habits after childbirth and beyond. You are allowed.

## Labour and Childbirth

## First Childbirth Experience

Even though it was ten years ago, I can still remember clearly going into labour with my eldest, my sweet son. For the specific details, I have also written it down in a little notebook. I've done it for all three of my children. I created this tradition of buying a little notebook for each of my children, so I can write down my thoughts and all the important first steps in the first years of their life but also remember each childbirth experience.

My first experience going into labour was on a Monday morning, early spring. I wake-up at six am, I can't sleep. My mind is busy, all sorts of thoughts cross my mind: I think about work, about the renovation work being done in our country home, about labour and how it will go … I was in a very strange and restless state of mind as if my intuition or higher self was alert and telling me to get ready.

I get-up and read for a while to try and find sleep. I get-up to go to the loo and notice I lose something that looks like the 'famous' mucous plug. When I now think about it, I knew something was happening, my intuition was trying to get my attention but I was not aware of it at the time. I finally go back to sleep when my husband gets up for work.

An hour later, I feel water running down my legs; my water broke! I try calling my husband who doesn't answer as he was still driving his motorbike to work.

I immediately call Anna Roy, my midwife, who is really excited and tells me "It's great, get ready, have breakfast and leave for the hospital!" I manage to get hold of my husband who immediately comes back. Meanwhile, I have a shower, get dressed, close my maternity suitcase. I'm ready but I am feeling really nervous.

I can't believe this is it, that I'm going to give birth and meet my son! I was slightly trembling, feeling more and more scared, I call my mum to let her know.

When my husband arrives, he tries to find a taxi; being in the centre of Paris on a busy Monday morning, it was tricky, but we finally managed. During all this time, I have no pain and couldn't feel any contractions. I wasn't quite sure when it was going to start.

When we arrived at the maternity, Anna Roy had warned everyone and they were waiting for me. Valentine, a midwife takes me to a birth room, examines my cervix and puts the monitoring around my belly. My cervix is only two cm open and I have no contractions. This was ironical knowing my contractile uterus condition and after being so careful during the last three months.

My baby was doing fine, the heartbeat was regular. Anna comes to see me which reassures me and gives me the confidence I needed.

After two hours of monitoring, they decide to put me in a regular room to see how things evolve. Shortly, this will be the room where I will be a new mum with my baby. Anna tells me to go and have lunch, and walk around the hospital corridors as much as possible to help accelerate the contractions. My husband and I are surprised with the way things are going. We felt no stress, we felt good.

I even was so lucky to have my favourite pasta dish with pesto at the cafeteria! The little gifts from the Universe, if you are aware, they exist much more than you think.

We walk in the corridors all afternoon. I had the pressure of making it happen naturally because since my water broke in the morning, I didn't have much time ahead of me to avoid the oxytocin injection the next morning. At the end of the afternoon, I rest in my room, have a meal and watch a film with my husband.

I'm not into the film and I am desperately hoping and talking to my son that it has to happen tonight if we want the chance of doing it by ourselves. Little did I know, thirty minutes later, I start feeling pain in my lower back and very quickly, I start to have painful contractions. I walk around the room, try to breathe, try to handle the pain but I apprehend the next contraction so much.

I am very tense, and I grasp onto anything I can while the contraction is at its summum. We call the nurse to go down to the birth room, but she looks at me and says: "No, I don't think you're ready, you can wait a bit more."

Inside my head I'm like: "I'm going to lose it!" I'm just trying to manage the pain as much as I can but inside, I am screaming. I used the courage I had left and I waited a little more until I couldn't take it anymore.

It's eleven-thirty pm and my cervix is only four cm open. I'd like to have a bath to help with the pain but when I get up, I lose quite a lot of blood and Nathalie, the midwife, prefers to do an epidural. It takes a while until the anaesthetist arrives; I'm trying to handle the pain as much as I can. Installing the epidural was epic, as it was almost impossible to stay still with the explosive and frequent contractions.

Once done, I fairly rapidly feel some relief but only on one side! After changing sides, it kind of balanced itself out and the pain disappeared, but I feel the sensations and I can move my legs! At one point, when the anaesthetic was working on one side, I couldn't feel my left leg. I can remember how frightening that felt. How are we supposed to give birth, listen to our body if we are completely numb?

My bladder being full, I had to empty it before giving birth, but it was impossible because the anaesthetic blocks all my natural sensations, including weeing! After a while, they decide to empty my bladder with a catheter. It's a really uncomfortable and very disagreeable experience yet being painless.

I am rapidly nine cm open, which makes me think that with all that waiting, I could have done it without an epidural but it's my first childbirth, I don't know what to expect and I am frightened.

Being in a natural birth friendly maternity, the lights were dimmed, and a wonderful nurse gave me great tricks on how to sit (not lie down), fold my legs (no stirrups) and slightly join my knees together in order to open the way for my baby.

By folding your legs and joining your knees slightly together, you are opening your pelvis, so opening the delivery path.

My baby is pushing so hard but it's that moment where you can't push yet, it is a very destabilising moment. Luckily, it doesn't last long and I can finally push. I am very concentrated and determined to do my very best to make things go fast and well. The nurse helps me to know when and how to push. A miracle technique: when the contraction arrives, breath out to go with the contraction, pull your knees slightly together while pushing.

Unfortunately, my contractions are slowing down and my baby is halfway there, so we have to hurry. Nathalie, the midwife, injects some oxytocin to speed things up. I can feel everything, it burns; my baby was coming through. When I think I still need to push, Nathalie asks if I want to catch my baby. "What? He's out? It's over?"

I take my baby between my legs and put him on my tummy, what a relief! My baby is here! What an amazing, unique, powerful, overwhelming, beautiful moment.

My baby boy cries a bit but calms down very fast once against by breast. The placenta now has to come out and again I feel a lot of apprehension. "Will it hurt? Will it take long? Will it all come out?" Finally, after pushing twice, it's all out. My husband is almost out too with all this pressure and emotions. The nurse cuts the umbilical cord for my husband, which is very well in the end.

Quite frankly even up and standing, I don't think my husband would have enjoyed the experience.

I can't think, I can't even really talk, I am somewhere else, somewhere between heaven and earth with my baby. Nathalie needs to sow a superficial tearing. I'm not too reassured but it all goes well. I don't care about the discomfort, I have my baby in my arms. Finally, he is here; it feels like a lifetime wait and battle.

We stayed two hours and a half in the birth room, at six-thirty am, we finally all go up in the room. My husband goes home to get some sleep. I wanted him to stay with us but there wasn't a real bed, and he was really needing the rest. I wonder if it's not harder for the fathers who experience birth from outside.

And as a new mother, I think of my family's needs first. I didn't know at the time that it was only the beginning of the path to devotion. That night, I didn't sleep, I stayed up admiring my blond, 3.300kg sweetest baby boy.

## Second Childbirth Experience

My second baby, my darling girl, arrived as a wonder. With this pregnancy, I worked literally until the very last minute. I was managing my company alone and I had taken the difficult decision to sell my company and take some time to look after my two children.

The last month of pregnancy was very stressful and tiring. I was negotiating the sale, discussions back and forth with the lawyers and accountants, plus all the daily micromanaging of the company and transition details I had to handle. On the morning of the day I gave birth, I signed the termination of the lease for my office.

I can remember clearly one of the parties joking and saying: "Take it easy, we don't want you giving birth in the meeting room," little did they know.

So, after this long day, I felt the urge to relax and let go. I was extremely happy to go to my yoga class down the street which was every Tuesday evening. After an hour of exercise, I get-up and stretch against the wall and I feel warm liquid run down my legs. During the whole class I could feel my body was not as usual, I suddenly realise what is happening.

I could feel different sensations in my body, it was reacting to the postures in an unknown way. So, I waited a little bit standing up and I feel water run down my legs again, much more abundant this time. At this moment, I knew it, my baby girl was coming and she would be with us the very same evening. I discreetly get out of the classroom and go to the toilet.

My waters is so abundant, that I keep pulling out layers of paper towels to limit the damage. I go to the classroom door and discretely call Sophie; the other mummies are in relaxation. I tell her "My waters just broke." She is in shock and doesn't know what to do.

She asks me if I need help or if she can call my husband. I tell her in a very calm and confident voice, "No worries, Sophie, I will walk home. I am around the corner." On the way home, I call my husband and tell him that our baby girl is coming that he and my son should slowly get ready. I also call my mum so she can come and help us to look after our son.

This peace, confidence was coming from within, from somewhere unexpected and that had been woken-up and nurtured during the yoga class.

When I get home, my husband is preparing diner. We tell our son very calmly that his little sister is going to arrive and that it is time for Mummy and Daddy to go to the hospital. My suitcase is not entirely packed, I wasn't expecting to give birth so soon. My husband quickly helps me pack everything. He suggests I take a shower before we go, but I want to keep this state of relaxation as long as possible that I think "Hey! Let's have a bath!"

So, I have a nice, not too warm bath to continue to maintain this serenity I am in. In the bath, I breath in and out calmly and let the contractions come without resisting them, just letting it flow. My husband brings me a bowl of quinoa and a glass of water, just enough to have the right amount of energy and be hydrated for the delivery. The contractions are getting more and more painful.

I don't want to wait too long and risk giving birth in the car on the way to the hospital so I get ready to leave. All three of us walk out of our apartment in central Paris heading for our car which is in our carpark nearby. While I am waiting in the street for my husband and son to get the car, I am on the phone with my accountant for the sale of my company and concentrating on the pain and contractions. Woman multitasking in action!

In the car on our way, I call my sister to let her know. She is so surprised how things are unfolding and how calm I am. My husband drops me off in from of the hospital and goes to park the car. I waddle my way up alone to the emergency waiting room and ring on the emergency bell.

I wait there for a while doing my yoga postures, stretching against the walls, breathing, stretching my arms up to the sky. I am in big pain, but I am in flow with my body. I had emptied myself (bladder and intestines) twice during the whole bath/waiting room period. I mention these details because it showed me how amazing the body is and how every detail is so perfectly and precisely orchestrated for birth. This, however, only when you are in tune and listen to your body. Sophie and her yoga classes taught me so much on that level.

Shortly after, the nurse, my husband and my son arrive in the waiting room. I am so relaxed and calm that the nurse didn't believe me when I told her I was going to give birth. She brings me to a birth room, tells me to do a urine test and to wait. Meanwhile, my contractions are getting closer and very painful, but I work with them and I do my yoga 'perineum expire' exercises.

I also talk to my baby, telling her that we are in this together and that we can do this. My mum arrives to pick-up my son and my husband leaves the room. The nurse puts the monitoring on my belly, so I now have to lay down. I take off my dress and underwear to be prepared, as I feel deep down it was going to happen very fast.

The midwife examines me and says my cervix is six cm open. She tells me how well I am managing the contractions and that she is very impressed. It gives me the strength to continue without any sedative or epidural. The pain quickly gets very hard to endure and my husband still isn't back.

Suddenly, I have one extremely painful and powerful contraction. I am sweating, I feel like vomiting, it's like my whole body is just taking over. I am alone in the room, or I prefer to say 'we' were alone with my baby, but we were managing extremely well. The nurse comes back to check on me, another awful contraction arrives. In the intensity of the pain, I ask for the injection, but the midwife is back and she says, "No time, the head is here."

My husband finally arrives. I am sitting on the edge of the birth table in a sweat when another contraction arrives and this time, a powerful force that came from my whole being pushed my baby down. I am ten cm open, and it's time to follow the uncontrollable push. I lay down on the table put my arms up behind me like in my yoga classes, breath and push the best I can.

I am concentrated, I am calm, I am confident. The midwife tells me I am doing an excellent job, that I am managing extremely well.

I push three times, the last push was for my baby's shoulder. The sensation is so powerful and so natural. It is amazing to be fully awake, conscious, and connected to the natural course of the delivery. I push one more time and my baby girl is here. She immediately cries as if she was telling me, "We've made it. I'm scared, where are you Mummy."

The midwife puts her on my tummy and my baby stops crying in an instant. How wonderful, how magical, how proud I am, in awe, I gave birth all by myself! I feel these waves of happiness, love and divine feminine power. This was when something changed in me forever. My perception of pregnancy, of childbirth, of pain, of my inner powers, of life.

This first breath of new life we took in unison with my daughter, where time was suspended, was as if my whole body and soul got a glimpse of the invisible, the life force we all have, and that is all around us.

My dream delivery came true! I remember saying to myself, "It was so amazing! I could do it again tomorrow."

We all experience this bliss when we give birth, but I guess I embraced it consciously. I had abandoned myself completely to the natural laws of my body and to my inner knowledge. I consciously perceived something, I now want to share with you.

## Third Childbirth Experience

My third miracle, just like her personality, arrived steadily, confidently, determined and with poise. It started on a Monday (again) at nine-thirty pm. I was lying on the couch talking to my husband while I had regular and close contractions but with no sensations nor pain whatsoever. Again, I knew deep inside I was slowly going into labour, but I didn't trust my intuition having no pain, I thought it was a kind of 'pre-labour' phase.

I called my sister who lived close by at the time just in case. My intuition getting stronger, an hour later, we ask her to come and sleep over and watch the children in case we need to leave in a rush. My sister arrives at eleven pm, but my contractions have stopped, so at eleven forty-five pm we all go to bed.

I immediately fall asleep but I am woken-up by a painful contraction at twelve-thirty am, then soon after, a second painful contraction arrives. I am about to wake-up my husband when I hear a huge burst sound and feel my waters soak the bed. The sound was very impressive, a very clear message we had hurry to the hospital.

I wait in our building hallway while my husband gets the car from the carpark. The contractions are getting more and more painful and at a very fast pace. It's twelve-fifty am, we are on our way, but the Bluets maternity hospital is far away, on the other side of Paris. Luckily, it's in the middle of the night and there is no traffic on the very busy and famous Parisian 'périphérique' highway.

The journey seems long and each bump on the road is becoming a torture. We arrive at the maternity and I am handling my contractions well with my breathing and focus but I can feel that I am going to give birth very soon. In the lift, I wonder how I am going to be able to wait in the emergency waiting room, the pain is getting unbearable.

We ring on the emergency bell, and I wait while my husband leaves to park the car. My contractions are getting intolerable, and my baby is now pushing to come out. I am starting to feel very anxious because of all the warnings I got during my pregnancy for my praevia cervix condition. I was afraid of strong bleeding and of an emergency C-section.

A midwife arrives. I explain in a hurry my praevia situation and tell her I need the epidural for safety reasons. She takes me to a room which is just an exam room. An interne arrives and asks me to do the traditional urine test and tells me she is going to put the monitoring belt on. I tell her, "There is no time for any of that, I am giving birth!"

During the waiting time and the short period of time in the exam room, I was handling the pain with my 'perinée expire' stretching and breathing techniques. But now, I was in such pain, the contractions were giving me no time to rest.

Within a fraction of a second, the interne lies me down, exams my cervix and tells me my cervix is nine and a half cm open, not to say ten cm. She calls her colleague in a rush, and this is when time starts to speed-up and that the events start to get intense.

The midwife who arrives, presents herself: "I'm Juliette, it's time to push!"

I was like "Yes, I know! and what? We are calling our daughter Juliette!" Nothing is a coincidence in life; life is so magical in every way. I pushed about four times, and my Juliette was born at one-fifty am, one hour after we had left home. Once more, no words can express how I feel and the beauty of the moment.

It's just like you are somewhere between earth and heaven where no time exists. Where you physically meet this little soul, whom you are in charge of for the rest of your life.

My little girl is on my tummy and immediately starts to breastfeed. The midwife and nurse keep me on observation because of the bleeding. I had expulsed the placenta but I was still bleeding quite a lot. My baby is now with her dad. The nurses and the midwife were clearly in disagreement on some procedure undertakings. They were discussing in front of me, as if I wasn't in the room, that my situation was concerning and that I may need a blood transfusion.

They were debating on my blood type, the need to warn the emergency service and reanimation wing. All this time, I was in a basic exam room on a very hard and basic exam table. My husband always jokes about it now, that I gave birth in the supply cupboard. After a while, they tell me they need to do a spinal anaesthesia in order to do a manual uterine revision to stop the bleeding.

The anaesthesia works immediately, and I am completely paralysed. It's a scary feeling, your brain is giving the command to move your legs, but nothing happens. They carry me on a stretcher and install me in a birth room. The doctor arrives. I try my best to be the most relaxed as possible, all goes well. The sensation of a hand in your uterus, right up to your ribs is extremely uncomfortable but it was painless.

The doctor also did a three cm stich were I usually tear during childbirth. My husband quickly joins me with our little girl. She is calm and peaceful on her father's chest, they are both skin to skin. I now wait to get my legs back. It was very long, and I was really starting to panic, "What if I never feel my legs again?"

Meanwhile, Juliette, the midwife, examines my Juliette and puts her in her first onesie. My husband starts to feel really weak, so two nurses take care of him.

At five-thirty am and after finally getting my legs back, we head for our room, where this time, my husband stays with us and sleeps next to us on a mattress. I can finally relax, breastfeed and in awe look at my beauty. We wake-up at eight-thirty am, yes two hours of sleep, and we have some breakfast. My husband being there, I can have a shower and wash my hair. Bliss! I can't express how good it feels.

It's really important to be able to take care of yourself right after birth and have some support after everything you have been through. We don't know this enough and most of all we don't feel legitimate. You deserve to rest and be fully supported.

## The Tools for Pain Management and Birth

The idea of giving birth can be terrifying for some of us, and most often, we don't talk about it. For others, it doesn't seem that scary, but they would like to know how to give birth more naturally or more in tune with their needs.

I am going to start this subject by being a bit harsh, maybe to create a reaction inside of you. If you lie there in the labour room, waiting for the contradictions to get closer and stronger, what do you think will happen? Yes, you will end-up only be focusing on the pain, and I can assure you, it is going to be unbearable. But this is what epidurals are for, right?

Yes, an epidural will cut you off from all sensations and connection to your body and baby. You will be there, but at the same, you won't. You will feel scared, anxious and you will hope all this is over fast enough. Most of the time, an epidural will slow down the contractions, making them less efficient, and making the labour time much longer.

You will then probably get an oxytocin injection to get things to speed up a little. It will help, but it will still make the contractions weaker, and since you are not feeling anything, it will be hard to push. Luckily, the doctor, midwife and nurse are here to guide you and do 60% of the work. This is harsh, right? But it is true.

As I have already shared, I have experienced both types of childbirth and for experiencing it in my body and mind, I can fully and confidently advance what I am saying. Now just like any other well-being or motivational advice we are told to work on now days, to give birth to a human being asks for courage. The courage to go in that labour room and be there with yourself and say: "I am going to give birth, I am calling on my power to give birth to my baby."

Let's be honest, when you go to the hospital, usually it's when you are sick or something is wrong. The sanitised smells, the colours, the neon white lights, doesn't help you feel relaxed and confident. The protocols when you arrive to give birth are numerous and it makes it very difficult to connect to yourself and to reappropriate your body. Your intention is where your focus goes and with all this trivia and this scary environment, it's hard to not to focus on it.

So, whether you eventually need an epidural or other medical assistance, the mindset and trust in yourself is essential.

Easy to say, how can this be done? How can we gain the trust in our own capabilities? And how can we access our inner strength?

My first answer is knowledge of your own body. It may sound like a huge and vast subject but ultimately you only need to know a few things and put them into application with repetition, to start understanding your body and how you can actually work with it. You can learn to 'embody your body' and handle giving birth by yourself and less medically assisted.

By preparing your body physically with persistence, you will just know what to do. Deepak Chopra says it well: "Knowledge of any kind gets metabolised spontaneously and brings a change in awareness from where it is possible to create new realities." Here could it be giving birth naturally?

The click for me was at my prenatal yoga classes with Sophie Colombié, in Paris. I had been practicing with her for a while when suddenly, during one class, I realised that with just some of the postures and breathing techniques, I could give birth fully aware of what was going on and what to do.

There were several breathing techniques allied to some stretching positions that with repetition gave me, in an instant, the confidence in my body and my capabilities to give birth. I could actually give birth naturally without an epidural and with trust in myself rather than with apprehension, fear and stuck in the pain.

My second answer is to train your mind. Did you know that while meditating, serotonin and oxytocin hormones are released in the body? The very hormones we need to give birth! I thought this was crazy when I found out. While they are naturally released in the body during labour, can you imagine if you help your body produce more or in a more powerful way?

Now of course, I am not saying we should meditate in the birth room like a yogi. But you can enter a state of mind and conscious connection that allows the calmness and clarity of meditation. You can train your mind while you are pregnant, to love yourself, trust yourself. You can learn how to love and trust yourself, by taking care of yourself.

To do so, taking the habit of meditating and implementing other self-care tools I share in the book, will create this mindset you need to give birth.

# Notions of Your Body to Understand for Labour and Childbirth

### Retroversion of the pelvis

To retrovert your pelvis is a simple yet very important notion to remember. You will need it for the next steps and when you give birth.

To grasp the idea you need to try. Stand-up and position your seat bones towards the ground and slightly towards the front. Bring your pubis forward and slightly upwards. If you put your hands at the bottom of your back, you will feel that your back is flat. Your tummy will be less prominent, and your baby will be brought at the back of your uterus.

### Breathing: Understanding How Your Diaphragm Works

As you probably know, breathing during labour and childbirth is primordial. For my first baby, the prenatal classes where they explain how to breath during labour and childbirth, was like watching a boring documentary. I got out of the class just as I came in, clueless.

One of the things you need to know is how your diaphragm works. When you know that when you inspire your diaphragm goes down and when you exhale your diaphragm goes up, you've understood most of it. You feel the contrary in your body because you feel the lungs being filled-up and emptied with air, but not your diaphragm going up and down.

What is really happening is that when you inspire your lungs fill-up and your diaphragm goes down and when you exhale your lungs empty while your diaphragm goes up.

Why does it help to know this when you give birth? When you understand this notion and visualise it while pushing, you really start pushing, you are really understanding how your body works and you are working with it.

When you feel a contraction arrive, you must prepare yourself. You take a deep breath in; when you are doing so, you are pushing down with your diaphragm, you are opening the way and pushing down your baby. When the contraction is at its strongest, you exhale out long and slow, you are efficiently pulling-up your diaphragm which contracts your uterus and all your rib muscles and continues with full strength the descent and expulsion of your baby.

This is only one of the notions you must understand. As I said, you need the combination of notions, to fully follow the natural process of childbirth. The other notions are the following.

### Stretching, Movement and the Three Postures for Pain Management

From experience of two natural births without epidurals, I only used three very simple stretching exercises again and again during labour. I learnt these postures with Sophie Colombié in my yoga classes. I found that repeating them again and again helped me concentrate on my body and sensations, without any effort, basically without overthinking.

It allowed me to work with my body, release some pain and connect with my baby. It's like saying a big 'YES' to your body and to childbirth!

## Movement

I realised most recently and with many years of practicing different types of yoga, that the notion of movement is so important. When we think about it, everything in life is movement. Nothing is fixed and yet we tend to think with fix ideas and images. We tend to move through life block by block rather than with movement and intention.

Specifically, during labour and childbirth, movement is primordial. While your body is preparing, synchronising each specific detail to give birth, you can do the same and accompany the process.

If you close your eyes, while there is no pain, find some kind of calmness and connection in your body. Listen to your corporal sensations, from your skin, to your muscles, to your bones. Now try moving, without thinking or with self-consciousness, just move in ways that feel natural, spontaneous, and relieving.

Like water, make gentle waves, you are fluid like a liquid. Stretch your arms if you feel the need; bend, twirl, undulate your body.

When a contraction comes, rather than blocking out the pain or tensing-up in apprehension, prepare for one of the postures I explain here below. Remember, everything is movement. Feel, move, and follow the process, you can do this. Repeat the cycles from moving and connecting when there is no pain, to focusing with a posture during the contraction.

Feel free to adapt and change your cycles to your needs.

**Position one: Upward forward fold**

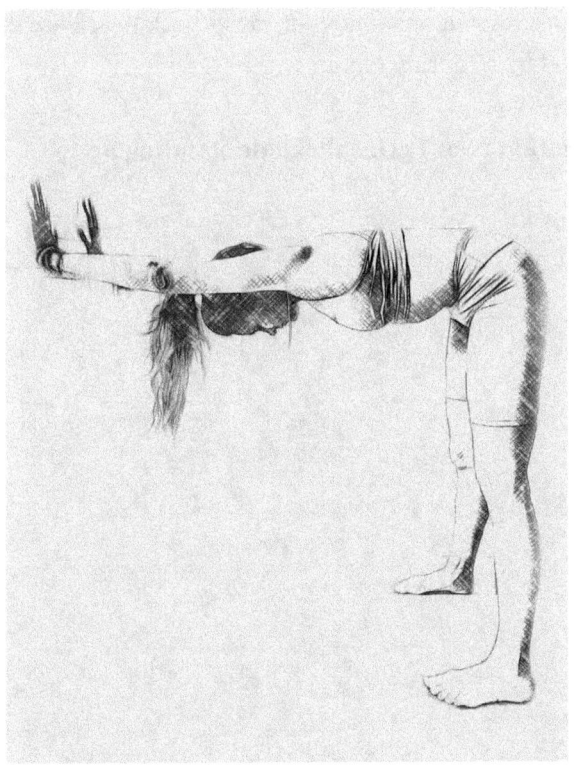

The first position is to find a wall, bend over 90° with your hands flat on the wall, palms flat and fingers open like a star. Your hands must be at shoulder level, your arms straight pushing against the wall as if you wanted to push the wall away from you.

Your legs must be straight and strong, your feet under your pelvis/hips (pelvis width). When a contraction arrives, take a deep breath in and just before the contraction gets strong and painful you breathe out all the air, long and slow through your lips. Push your hands against the wall, arms strong and push your legs in the ground. You are stretching your muscles and opening your lower back to release the pain localised there during labour.

**Position two: Perineal exhale standing up**

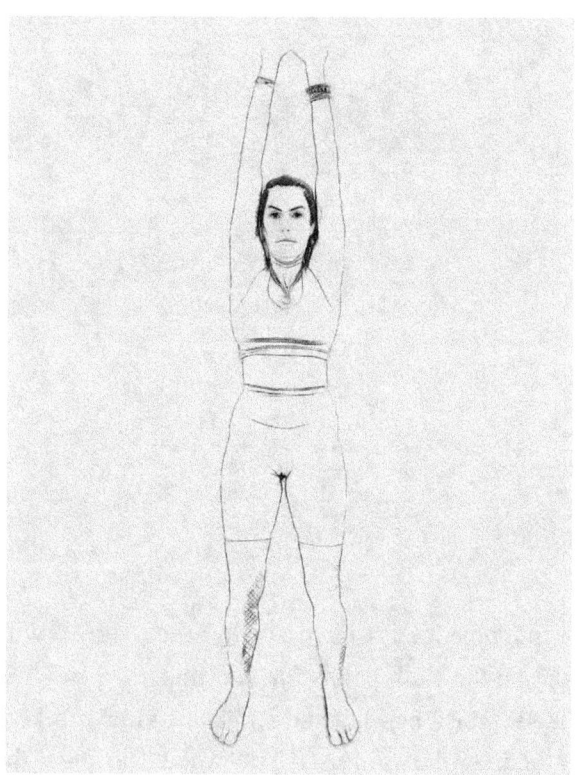

The second one is very similar, you are doing it standing-up without any support. When you feel a contraction arrive, put your hands in the air, arms straight, hook your index fingers together, place your legs hip wide and breath in deep. This is when you retrovert your pelvis. Remember, push your seat bones and pelvis forward to flatten your lower back. When the contraction gets strong and painful, breath out long and slow, and while doing so push your hands in the air as if you were stretching to the sky.

You are protecting your lower back, releasing some pain, and opening the way for your baby. I want you to make a sound while breathing out, do it, don't feel silly doing so, just listen to your needs. Making a sound can help you put the intention in the breathing and feel it more powerfully.

### Position three: Perineal exhale lying down

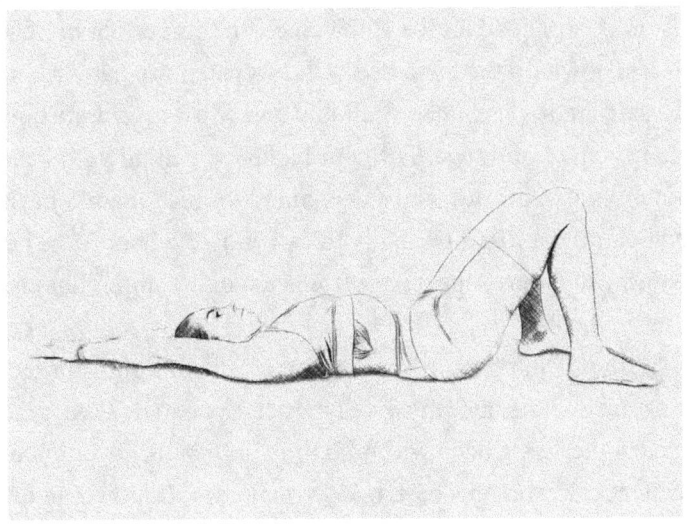

The third one is also the position you use to give birth. Lie down on the birth bed, bend your knees, put your feet flat on the bed, width slightly larger than your hips. Pull your hands up behind you as if you wanted to touch the top of the bed. Your arms straight, hook your index fingers together and when you feel a contraction arrive, inspire deeply.

When the contraction is there, breath out deep and slow, pull up your hands and stretch your arms as if you wanted to touch the bed. While doing so, retrovert your pelvis by pushing your feet in the mattress. The retroversion of your pelvis will happen naturally this way. When the contraction is over, let go, relax and breath normally.

## Positioning: The Position for a Physiological and Fast Birth

The position I used to give birth was the last stretching posture I explained above with some extra important notions.

Lie down on the birth bed. I did so when my baby's head was starting to push uncontrollably and when my whole body was in a state of trance. Put your hands up behind your head, stretch your arms out as if you wanted to push the top of the bed behind you. This time, if you can, grab the bars of the bed behind you or any other support you have. It's important your arms are active.

Rather than opening your legs wide and putting your feet-up as the doctors and midwives may tell you to do, keep your feet on the birth bed, width slightly larger than your hips. Then most but not the least, bring your knees slightly together, so inwards.

By bringing your knees together, you are opening the bottom of your pelvis from one to two centimetres, so opening the path for your baby. This is a lot when it comes to pushing out a baby. On the contrary, when you open wide your legs you are closing your pelvis. This is called nutation and counter nutation.

When you add the breathing, the stretching and the leg/knee positioning, you are creating a path for your baby, you are working with your body, you are surrendering to the amazing process of childbirth.

**Trusting: Connect with yourself and with your baby**

I wasn't meditating at the time, so even with that important aspect lacking in my life at the time, I managed to connect somehow to my inner strength and with my baby.

By applying what I explained above, it put me in a state of relaxation, in a state of trust and confidence. I was reappropriating my body and capabilities. I was aware of the pain, but I accepted it; I went with it. When you do this, it is much more endurable, and by the way, we are made to survive it.

We tend to think that everything is separate in the world, that everything has boundaries. But your baby is inside of you, your baby is with you and she or he is listening to you, feeling your energy and vibrations.

If you put your hands on your tummy and talk to your baby, tell your baby you are going to do this together, that you are a team and that you are ready. Then you jump into the experience that is going to happen together, no matter what you do. So, embrace it with your baby, and meet her or him on the other side in a way no words can describe.

## Home childbirth

If you have the right training and the right person to accompany you, giving birth at home is possible. Know that it is not a decision to take lightly. Unless all means of security for mother and baby are assured, you must be aware you are taking a risk. Each woman and baby are different, and anything can arise within a second. It is not worth the glory. Most of the time, we have fixed ideal images in our mind or rigid expectations of how we want to give birth.

Natural childbirth with no epidural is not a trendy thing to do but rather a true belief, a real quest from within to reconnect with your feminine strength and powers. It's also about confidence and confidence comes with knowledge that brings self-trust and true capability. Knowledge comes with training, and you must prepare for birth at home just like an athlete would prepare for a major competition.

Basically, you must be fully prepared, if this is something you really want to experience. Learn to know your body and how to work with it, with prenatal yoga exercises. Get to know your perineum and pelvis, how it works during labour. Get to know yourself in the calm of meditation.

Have a doula or a trained prenatal accompaniment, who will be there by your side. And of course, the last but not the least, have a certified midwife or nurse for a secured and smooth home childbirth.

We will get to normalising home childbirth in the future, we will get there but we need the training first. We must show the right example for this path to be followed correctly.

## SOS 1st Months

When baby is here, like all first-time mums, we have no idea whatsoever about having a baby and we just 'do', out of the blue, instinctively what we think is best. Most of the time, we are just coping one day at a time. And you know what? This is great; we should trust ourselves more.

When my baby was born, I was more in the 'doing' and 'reacting' to the situations that would come up with my baby, rather than being in the 'feeling' and 'responding' in the moment with confidence. Being exhausted with a lack of many hours of sleep doesn't help the mind to be clear and to be in tune with our soul.

I love being a mum. I think it's one of my most important paths in life, to carry little souls and bring them into this world. If I could, I wouldn't stop having babies! (I am giggling when I write this.) I also think I experienced difficult situations around motherhood, to be able to learn and grow from them and then share with the collective.

I always try to think out of the box and question what is taken for granted. In motherhood, it is very easy to get carried away and follow what we are told to do and what society tells us what is best. Just like Deepak Chopra says: "Question dogma, question ideology (…) it is only by questioning what people hold to be true, that we can break through the hypnosis of social conditioning."

The tips I am about to share are the results of my struggles, and the wonderful solutions I discovered or was given. The tips are effective and nurturing. Nurturing for you, for your baby, and it always carries the fundamental question: "How can we, mother and baby, go through this transformational period mindfully and the most comfortably possible?"

o **How Do I Feel?**

Surprisingly, I added this section when my book was almost finished. One evening, I was watching a film of a young mother who was in her first month of postpartum. She was sitting on her couch crying and just feeling horrible. It struck me! How could I not talk about this feeling and period after birth more in depth?

I have experienced it myself with my first baby and I can relate feeling so sad and lonely. I remember being at the hospital two days after giving birth and just crying in my hospital bed, all alone, feeling basically depressed. I felt so guilty to feel this way. I was meant to be happy, thrilled, excited to finally have my baby. And there I was, feeling sad and awful in my body.

Now many factors explain this state and we don't all experience it. I know that I hadn't slept for like three nights, and that the sudden drop of hormones and other personal reasons got the best of me. The most important thing to know, is that IT IS OK. It is normal, you are not alone, and IT WILL PASS.

The most important thing is to trust it will pass, that it is safe to feel like this. It is also important to be surrounded and supported by your husband or partner, your family or your friends.

Don't hesitate to call for the midwife or nurse, they can also provide support.

I love what the mother of the young woman in the film told her: "There is something when you get pregnant that no one talks about. It is that you mourn a little a bit. You mourn the person you used to be; no matter how much you want to become a mum, you're never not going to be one again. That is a huge brain adjustment. You are letting go of the old self."

So, whether it's the hormones, the lack of sleep or loneliness, this is so true. This notion itself is more than enough to make you feel sad and down. But know, that you will slowly feel normal again in your body and in your heart. Therefore, the tools I share in this book are so important because they show you the path and provide the support you need to feel YOU again.

A new you, yes as a mum, but a whole new you again. This is the best 'you' in your life.

o   **What Is Bonding?**

What does bonding mean? The definition of bonding is the intense attachment that develops between parents and their baby. Ten years ago, I didn't hear anything about bonding, and it wasn't a notion that was of great interest. Today, there are more and more studies that show how important it is for babies and their emotional and social development.

We all naturally, in some way, bond with our newborn, we don't really think about it. We feel love for our baby, we take care of our baby, and we meet all of her/his needs.

However, bonding does go further and it is more subtle than we think. Today, I clearly realise I didn't truly bond with my first child until three months of age. Something happened with my second child, where I got a glimpse of what bonding really meant at about three weeks of age. And with my third child, I did it deliberately after birth.

It's unfair in a way that it happened earlier for some and later for another. Maybe, but I always did my very best for each of my children; I loved them each just as much with all my heart. I have no regrets, as I was ignorant not unloving. And most of all, I am human and learning, we all are, and this is why it is not good or bad, it just is.

Let's be kind with ourselves. It's important not to judge ourselves too harshly in motherhood, otherwise it can give rise to unnecessary guilt and suffering. You are doing your best and it's impossible to give exactly the same to each of your children in an identical pattern. You are giving as much, but differently, in a unique way.

So bonding is seeing your baby, really seeing your baby as an individual, as a unique soul and personality. When you really see, you become one with your baby, it's this notion of oneness again. It is a powerful feeling that flows through your body, and it comes up with 'I truly know you' and you feel this unconditional love and knowing.

How can we bond? Eye contact is one of the first ways. We tend to take care of our baby by changing, washing, feeding, kissing, and getting on with our daily routine but we rarely take time to really stop and connect with our baby. With my first baby, I was very much in the doing and not in the feeling and connecting.

Having breastfeeding problems and a very agitated baby made it hard for me to appreciate the little moments. But one day, after my baby had breastfed and dreading the post feeding cries, I sat my baby up in front of me on my lap wanting to make my baby laugh (he was about three months old).

Something amazing happened, we looked at each other in the eyes and we started to smile and laugh in a true, authentic way. Something happened and I understood I hadn't been seeing my baby; I hadn't taken the time. I had a baby and I had problems; I was looking at the situation with separateness. Suddenly we were a WE, together, we bonded. It changed a lot of things after that.

For my second child, I was a happy and more confident mum (thank you experience) but one day, while I was getting ready to have a bath with my baby (about three weeks old), again something happened. We were both naked, skin to skin heading for the bathroom.

I held my baby in front of me in the happiness of the moment, and we looked at each other in the eyes, and boom! Connection; I met my baby. We had beaming smiles on our faces and a connection just flowed between us. I saw my baby differently after that; we had bonded.

For my third child, it was a few days after giving birth. I had returned home from the maternity. It was evening. I was sitting on the sofa with my baby on my chest, breathing and smelling my baby's hair. This time, tears started to run down my face and a strong feeling of pure love just flowed between us. The bonding was through the contact, the smell, the presence in the moment. I had met my baby.

Touch and massaging are another way to bond with your baby. You can do skin to skin contact moments at home on your sofa or on your bed. The first weeks of life is the best timing for skin to skin bonding. Your baby sleeps a lot and needs your warmth and smell.

Massaging is another wonderful bonding moment once your baby is one month of age. I give massage tips further on in the book. Before one month of age, it is good to start an introduction to massage with caresses. Your baby needs touch, movement and love to grow in a cocoon that feels safe.

When your baby is over a month, you can start the real massage movements. If you can, create eye contact with your child during the massage. If your baby avoids looking in your eyes, put your hands gently but firmly on the chest and connect through the touch. I massaged all three of my babies. With my second and third child, I used the IAIM (International Association for Infant Massage) movements.

I created a ritual where I would do a full body massage after the bath in the evening. It was our moment with my baby to relax and bond. Of course, sometimes baby is not in the mood or too hungry for a full massage, so I would just adapt to my baby's mood and do a shorter massage.

Your baby only lived through sensations of touch, movement and sound in your tummy. Your baby needs it during the first months of life outside the womb to feel safe and understood. Slowly but surely, your baby will grow out of this cocoon to feel confident and safe, pushed by the curiosity of discovering the world.

For some, it can be really hard to truly bond with their baby. Rather than feel guilty, ashamed, or live in denial, try and question yourself. What are you feeling inside when it comes to connecting with your baby? How do you feel? When?

Very often, it is because we are not taking care of ourselves, we are not loving ourselves. I recommend investigating inside and using the nurturing tools in this book to listen, soften and take care of yourself. If you feel you can't do it alone, which I insist, is perfectly OK, go and see a therapist. There is no shame in seeking for help, on the contrary it is a sign of higher consciousness and act of courage. I promise you it is worth it, don't waste time avoiding or pretending. Don't let old wounds or fear get in the way. You can feel proud of yourself and feel safe to open-up.

The relationship with your child is so important and it starts in the womb. Bonding with your baby allows you to have a relationship in connection with authentic love. Your child will need this all his/her life as an inner tool. It will allow your child to be one with his/her inner child. Your baby is securely loved and will always be able to trust him/herself no matter what happens in life.

o   **The Foundations of Breastfeeding**

Breastfeeding is tough for all mothers when we start. I have breastfed my three children and each time, the beginnings are very painful, and it can be stressful. I would get red nipples and huge cracks that would bleed and make breastfeeding a torture. The worst are the first days at the hospital, but it usually fades away after two or three weeks.

After that, feeding then becomes a precious moment of bonding with your baby.

Unfortunately, we don't have much help in hospitals or at home and we can easily feel discouraged in our new breastfeeding journey. For my first baby, I was extremely lost even though I did get some guidance at the hospital. There are many subtle details we are totally unaware of when we start breastfeeding. We can easily start to self-doubt and with the lack of knowledge, we end by giving-up.

I went to Leche League meetings in Paris to get the answers to my enquiries. I even saw a Leche League consultant at home to get the help I needed with my first baby. You must know that there is no such thing as 'your milk is not good enough, or rich enough' nor 'I am not good at this'.

Breastfeeding is the best thing you can offer to your child. It is scientifically proven to be the best. Yet, we shouldn't need science to prove anything, it comes from our body, how could it not be the best? Initially, alternatives like bottles and formula milk appeared for mothers who were physically or medically incapable of breastfeeding or for social beliefs in the upper classes of civilisation.

**Basic first step breastfeeding position**

Here are some tips that can help you when you start breastfeeding.

-   Make sure you are sitting-up comfortably with your back straight.

- Use your breastfeeding cushion or other cushion to support your baby, so you are not holding all the weight with one arm and shoulder.
- Make sure your baby is against you, in a position that is parallel on your lap (lying completely down on one side).
- Press on your baby's chin gently with your finger to make sure he/she opens the month wide enough to latch on.
- To do so, with your index finger and middle finger pinch the areola of your breast to help your baby latch on properly. Make sure your baby takes the whole areola and not just the nipple. If his/her mouth doesn't cover the whole areola of your breast, this is when it's gets extremely painful and when crevices quickly form.
- At the beginning, it is very common to have crevices, I've had it each time. And I can remember crying, it hurts so much. The only truly efficient ointment is Lanolin. It repairs and protects your nipple, it is edible and 100% safe for your baby.
- Do not use silicone breastfeeding nipples, it may be temping for the pain at first but it is almost sure that it will cause your breastfeeding journey to stop prematurely. Your baby can't latch on as well and it's really hard work for him/her to get enough milk out and it will create frustration.

Babies show signs of restlessness when they are frustrated and when there isn't enough milk flowing; pay attention to their signals. You will think your silicon nipples are wonderful at first and that it is the perfect solution to avoid the pain, but your milk production will slowly stop. And when the milk flow starts to slow down drastically, it is very difficult to get it abundant again.

I highly recommend you use Lanolin for the pain; it is natural, and you can find it in any pharmacy or online.

- If the pain lasts more than three weeks to a month, consult your paediatrician to make sure your baby doesn't have a tongue or lip-tie. A tongue and lip-tie are very common, and it can be corrected very easily. Do not worry, I hear you, it's painless for your baby and she/he will not remember anything about it.

**Milk supply**

When I started breastfeeding my first baby, the eldest of my three children, I had no idea what to expect. I was lucky to have a few guidelines given at the maternity hospital, during the following days after childbirth. This is one of the reasons I chose the 'Les Bluets' hospital in Paris. They are pro breastfeeding, the midwives and nurses guide you, encourage you and help you during the awkward first days.

However, I quickly found out this was not enough, and once I was at home, I rapidly realised something wasn't right since my baby was extremely restless while breastfeeding, and he would scream afterwards. I noticed I had a lot of milk, which I thought was a good thing. In general, we tend to think that a lot of something is better or good, but here it turned out to be a nightmare.

When my baby was three months old, I started to go to the Leche League meetings every Monday morning in Paris. I learnt many things about breastfeeding like 'strong ejection reflex', which I rapidly understood I clearly had. I tried to apply as many tips as possible at home, but my baby was still not comfortable.

Lea, from the Leche League in Paris, came for a private consultation at home to try and understand what the problem was. She finally understood after observing my baby while feeding. First of all, I did have too much milk. I needed to slow down the production, and secondly, my baby wasn't feeding long enough to get to the rich fatty milk he needed.

The following tips I am going to share are from my personal experience and research. I was given specific and efficient tools from the Leche League in Paris. The first facts date from ten years ago and some of the studies have evolved. All the information I share in this book has been checked on various platforms including the Leche League's website. After studying and comparing the facts, I found some differences and contradictions.

I have made sure the practical tips I share summarise the information so it is clearly understandable, but most of all that it assures the desired result: a smooth and happy breastfeeding journey for both mother and baby.

**Too much milk**

When you have too much milk, there are several things you can do to regulate your milk production:

1.  Control the 'strong ejection reflex'.

What's a 'strong ejection reflex'? Basically, it's when your milk comes out like a wild hose when you begin to breastfeed. The milk comes out too fast, too strong and far too much. Your baby can't follow the flow and will start choking, coughing and swallow too much air, which will create pain thus suffering and crying. Usually, your baby will quickly get agitated and even stop latching on because it is not manageable.

The way to calm this down is to empty your breast a little bit before your baby breastfeeds. Manually empty your breast so the flow is less strong, or use a hand pump or an electric pump. Extract a little bit of milk, just enough so the milk doesn't burst out anymore. Your baby will then find pleasure to latch on again with serenity and comfort, and will learn with time how to cope with the high flow of milk you tend to have.

2.   Slow down the production.

To slow down the production, you basically need to give one breast to your baby at each breastfeed. So, you only give one breast and then for the next feed, you switch breast and give the other side. You give one breast every other feeding. Doing so, you are entirely emptying your breast, leaving no left over. It will also take longer for your milk to reproduce.

You are basically sending a message to your body saying: "I have too much milk, you can slow it down." It will take from three to eight days for the production of your milk to find a new pace and balance, but it works as a charm.

**Not enough milk**

If you don't have enough milk, here is what you can do:

1.  Make sure you are not using any silicon nipples.

As mentioned before, silicon nipples are the worst thing when you start your breastfeeding journey. All the people I know who have used silicon nipples, have stopped breastfeeding after one or two months because they had no more milk and because their baby was complaining. Some, who realised before it was too late, suddenly saw their milk supply come back and sustain their baby again.

Important fact you must know that it is easier to slow down the production of your milk than to bring it back. Once you have very little milk or none, it is a tough task to get it back on flow again.

2.  Use both breasts at each breastfeed.

By using both breasts during each breastfeed, this time you are sending a message to your body saying: "I don't have enough milk, quickly make some more." You are stimulating the production of your milk. When you start to breastfeed, give one breast and then halfway through the feed give the other breast.

Each baby and breasts are different, so 'halfway' can be nine minutes or three minutes. You know what 'halfway' is for you, depending on the length of your breastfeeds. It can take between a week to fifteen days to find the right balance.

### The 'nineteen-minute magic'

After finding out, I had too much milk supply and learning how to slow down the production of my milk, things were a bit better, but my baby was still crying after each breastfeed. This is when I contacted a Leche League breastfeeding consultant, Lea, to come and help me at home.

I call it the 'nineteen-minute magic' because it was a total mental shift for me, it was so unexpected and surprising! When Lea told me that an average feeding lasts about nineteen minutes, I was in shock. My baby was done in seven minutes at the most! She explained that there are several phases during a breastfeed where the fat gradually builds-up in the milk, making the milk rich at the end of the feed.

She told me that the milk at the beginning of a breastfeed is much more watery, sweet in taste, but also hard to digest, and obviously not sustaining. So, because my baby wasn't breastfeeding long enough, he was not getting enough of the rich milk that comes at the end of an average nineteen-minute feed.

The two different types of milk during a breastfeed are known as:

The 'foremilk' and the 'hindmilk'.

- Foremilk is the milk at the beginning of a breastfeed, which is watery with less fat and high in lactose (milk sugar).
- Hindmilk which arrives is the second phase of a breastfeed, is richer and also called the 'crème' with a lower lactose amount.

These two milk notions are still used in many articles and official websites today, but the Leche League has changed the definition and the expertise on the matter. I was not told by Lea at the time probably because it was still unknown. But today, the Leche League mention on their website that the foremilk (watery milk), at the beginning of a breastfeed, is the result of a left-over of milk from the previous breastfeed and not because the foremilk has less fat.

Whatever the reason is, it is important to understand that your baby must have enough of the hindmilk, rich milk, to feel sustained and digest well without pain.

This is where understanding the notion of lactose overload will be very helpful.

**Lactose overload**

What's a lactose overload? To come back to my example, I was told that my baby was only getting the foremilk, which is less digestible and creates a lot of gastrointestinal (GI) issues. My mind was blown! I had too much milk AND my baby was only getting the 'watery' milk!

I finally understood why he was so frustrated, so upset, and why he would scream at the end of each breastfeed. He was suffering from what we call today a lactose overload or lactose imbalance.

To help you grasp this information, and help you apply the tips you need depending on your milk production, here is what a perfect breastfeed would look like:

- Baby properly latching on your breast.
- Baby breastfeeds on both breasts.

- Both breasts are completely drained after each breastfeed.
- Baby breastfeeds as long as possible (nineteen-minute magic).

Now as perfection doesn't exist, here is what it's really about. The importance isn't really the length in time, even though it is important your baby breastfeeds as long as possible to make sure she/he is fully sustained. My baby never breastfed for nineteen minutes, so do not worry if it's the case for you too. If your baby feeds for ten minutes, it doesn't mean he/she is only getting the watery foremilk.

What counts is the right quantity of milk and that your breast or breasts get entirely drained. This will allow the next feed to be with the new milk, with the right amount for your baby, and with a good foremilk/hindmilk balance.

It is the foremilk/hindmilk imbalance that creates a lactose overdose which will create gastrointestinal (GI) issues for your baby. It can also happen that the lactose overload causes similar symptoms to a lactose intolerance, which is very confusing, but the cause is different.

The digestion problems usually come from your baby consuming large volumes of breast milk. This may happen when you have an oversupply of milk, or when the time between the feeds is too long.

Like I already explained in the breastfeeding tips, if like me you have a lot of milk, empty your breast a bit before breastfeeding, and only give one breast. Make sure your baby drains your breast properly, so there is no more milk left.

Don't hesitate to help your baby release some air midway through the feeding, take a break, put your baby on your shoulder for a few minutes, you may hear a burp (or not) and then put your baby back on the same breast. If a bubble of air is creating discomfort, the chances are that your baby won't want to breastfeed any longer.

Last important factor, the length between feeds. There is no reason to create long gaps between feeds, like with formula-fed babies. I had this false idea because I had read and heard about it everywhere, that it was important to space feeds to three hours. So, I would gradually force my baby to wait an extra ten minutes at each feed, during several weeks to get to the three hours minimum.

Breastmilk is easily assimilated and digested, within twenty minutes, so there is no reason to create unnecessary frustration, which can be torture for your baby. This technique did not prove to be successful, and it didn't help me nor my baby.

Try and listen to the signs your baby is showing you. Once your milk production is suitable for your baby, things will get so much easier, and you won't even think about it anymore.

### Breast engorgement/mastitis

My first experience with mastitis was rather traumatic. I reassure you though, not the problem in itself, because there are great tips to help you handle it swiftly. And there are specialised breastfeeding doctors and midwives in case you can't manage it on your own. Meanwhile, I will provide straight forward and easy tips for breast engorgement before it becomes a mastitis.

I started to get mastitis with my first-born baby after several days of breast engorgement symptoms. My baby was three months old, when during a breastfeed, I realised I had a hard and painful breast and that the feeding didn't remove the discomfort nor did my breast get soft again. I tried to get my baby breastfeed that breast in priority in order to unblock the milk canal, but it didn't work.

As I was a new mum, tired and totally ignorant, I didn't realise it could become a problem until my breast got red patches. The pain during a breastfeed was unbearable and I started to have fever. In an emergency, I went to see my general doctor at the time, who had a look at my breast but clearly had no knowledge in breastfeeding whatsoever. He sent me to undertake other tests rather than treating me and suggesting me to see my midwife.

My experience with mastitis took huge proportions after this. I will highlight the physical and emotional violences that a new mother can endure with the medical field, later in the book in chapter 'Lets change things together'.

How to recognise a breast engorgement?

1. A very hard breast that doesn't get softer after breastfeeding.
2. Your breast is very painful until breastfeeding becomes unbearable.
3. Your baby may get frustrated and agitated on that breast because there isn't enough milk coming out.
4. You notice red patches on your skin and small lumps in your breast.
5. You feel feverish or have fever.

What can you do?

- First of all, you can try unblocking the milk canal manually in the shower. Massage your breast under hot water until you see a normal flow of milk and/or if your breast gets softer. You may have to do this several times, sometimes once is enough.
- For the pain, you can apply a cold compress or ice pack for about twenty mins. This helps for the pain and swelling, and it will allow the improvement of venous and lymphatic drainage.
- Express your milk with a manual or electric milk pump several times a day. This is the only thing that worked for me. I would rent an electric pump at my local pharmacy. Draining my breast between each breastfeed and expressing my milk just a little bit before I would breastfeed my baby worked for me.

  It asks for persistence, patience and courage, but it works. Expressing your milk much more often will stimulate your milk production, but once the canal is unblocked, then you will be able to go back to your normal pace and everything will get back into balance over a couple of days.

o **How to Survive Newborn Colic**

The first month with baby is usually surprisingly easy. You may jump to the ceiling when I say this, but from experience and taking in consideration that you have just brought a little human being into this world, the first month isn't the most difficult. Mostly, baby sleeps a lot and needs to recuperate from the exhausting and traumatic birth experience.

When your baby wakes-up, it's usually to breastfeed or to be changed. I've clearly noticed that the difficult period of ongoing crying or not knowing what my baby needs, is at the end of the first month. For all three of my children, it's as if they suddenly woke-up from a coma and faced the violent reality that they were not in my womb anymore.

This coincides with the maturing period of their intestines and activation of their digestive system. This is when we start talking about baby colics. Where baby suffers tremendously considering her or his little size and weight. The tummy pains are real and have the double effect of frightening our baby to the core.

This is the first time in their very existence that they feel this sharp and acute pain. Can you imagine how frightening it must be? When you don't know what it is or where it's coming from?

The only way for babies to express their pain and fear is to cry and cry as much as their little body can. One of the best ways to relieve baby's pain is to gently massage their tummy.

Sometimes, it's tricky if the umbilical cord hasn't fallen off yet, usually it has, but for some it can take longer. It can still be done with care with some gentle movements. I will share simple and effective massages that work for colics but also other beneficial massages for the whole body.

Another way to help your baby feel safe is by carrying her or him in a scarf or a physiological baby carrier. First of all, your baby will feel your warmth, your smell and hear your heartbeat. Your heartbeat, is like a calming song your baby heard and evolved with for nine months in your tummy. But also, being held tight and gently rocked around by your movements instantly reassures your baby; it brings your baby home.

o **What are the Evening Cries?**

This phenomenon is closely woven with the newborn colic. It doesn't appear with all babies, but it is extremely common (80% of babies). I understood these cry patterns with my second child, and it changes everything when you understand and know what to expect. The cries usually start around five pm or six pm in the evening and can last until twelve pm. Specialists say the anxiety starts with the nightfall.

Your baby seems desperate and extremely anxious and doesn't know how to calm down. These cries appear when your baby is about one month old (between six and eight weeks) and lasts for about a month. Then, you will notice a sudden stop where the evening cries just disappear.

If you are breastfeeding, your baby will ask to breastfeed very frequently, I noticed a frequency of every twenty minutes. It is one of the only ways your baby knows to feel secure and safe. The other tool, again, is carrying your baby with a scarf or physiological baby carrier. Your baby won't necessarily stop crying but it will make the cries less frantic, and most of all, it will give the warmth and love your baby needs.

It happened with my second baby that I had to walk around the living room non-stop until midnight. This was the peak of the evening cries, and it lasted a month. It was like my baby was in a trance and couldn't get out of it. I had started to understand that this was a normal phase, that I had to just go through it with my baby.

It doesn't make it less tiring nor stressful. However, knowing it is natural, that it doesn't last, and that you can help your baby by your warmth and presence, makes a huge difference in how you can navigate courageously and confidently through this experience.

For my third baby, I clearly knew what to expect and I felt much calmer and more confident. My baby felt it and I guess it made the experience more harmonious compared to my two first pregnancies. During this pivotal month, I breastfed my baby on demand; I carried and rocked my baby around the house. I didn't think, I just felt.

I also implemented in my baby's evening routine a bath and ended with a body massage before breastfeeding. This allowed my baby to relax and reconnect to the sensations of the body, the sensations of touch and movement. It's extremely important for your baby as these elements were all your baby knew in your tummy for nine months.

If your routine allows it, you can also have a bath with your baby. It is a lovely moment to bond with your newborn skin to skin, and to talk to her/him in a soothing atmosphere.

o **Introduction to Baby Massage**

I took baby massage classes with Sophie Colombié for my second child. Yes, Sophie again, my prenatal yoga teacher, she has many talents. Sophie showed me, and the other mums attending the course, the massage movements for babies from IAIM, the International Association for Infant Massage. The massage movements are the same as or inspired by the infant traditional Indian massages.

You can also find these massages in Frederic Leboyer's marvellous book *Shantala*, illustrated with an Indian lady and her baby. In Europe or the US, we are not very familiar and comfortable with massaging because it is not in our culture and traditions. In general, we are quite prude and bashful with our bodies and we are not aware of the benefits of the touching senses.

For your baby, it is a way to release tensions and relieve pain (colic), it is a way to relax and prepare for sleep and it is also a way to recognise and feel parts of the body your baby is not aware of. Where everything in the womb was feeling and sensation for your baby, massaging activates those soothing inherent memories.

**What you need to know for the massages.**

Usually, we wait until baby is one month of age before massaging. The first month your baby sleeps a lot and doesn't need an intrusive body stimulation. The end of the first month, also coincides with the moment where the umbilical cord falls off and the colic pains appear. The massage movements come in handy at this time.

However, knowing the importance of contact and warmth for your baby, the first month you can start an introduction to massaging with skin-to-skin cuddles and gentle strokes on your baby's skin before or after the bath or any other appropriate moment for your baby. Just listen to your intuition and your baby's signals.

Equipment wise, you will need a 100% natural vegetal oil, organic is better. You can either use coconut oil, almond oil, or if you don't mind the smell simply colza or olive oil. Heat the room before you start the massage, your baby must never feel cold. Do the massage on the floor on a towel with a waterproof changing mat underneath in case your baby does a wee.

Sit on your knees on the floor, place a yoga mat or cushion so you are comfortable. If you want to do it the Indian traditional way, Fréderick Leboyer shows in his book how you can massage your baby sitting on the floor, by using your legs as the support for the massage. Sit on the floor, your legs straight in front of you and place the waterproof changing mat and towel on your legs.

Place your baby facing you, on your legs lying down on his back, his feet towards you. I give instructions of left and right hand but if you feel comfortable the other way round, do what is most comfortable and natural for you.

**If your baby has tummy pains (colics)**

Usually when your baby brings up her/his legs towards the tummy while crying, and the tummy is very tense and hard, it's because of gas and colic pain. There are three exercises you can do to help relieve the pain. The exercises are from the IAIM course I did with my second baby in 2015.

1.  Water mill

First put both of your hands gently on your baby's tummy, breath in and out and relax. Look at your baby in the eyes.

With your left hand at the top of the belly and your right hand bellow the belly, alternatively gently press and swipe down, one hand after the other. Do so as if you were trying to get rid of some air stuck in the tummy going downwards. The gesture should be like a firm stroke. Repeat five to six times.

2.   The sun and moon

You are going to massage around the belly. One hand does a whole circle with your fingertips going clockwise. And the other hand does the same but only half a circle (from 10 to 5 clockwise).

3.   Knee push ups

Hold your baby's feet both in one hand and gently push the knees towards your baby's abdomen, naturally bending your baby's knees. Stay six seconds with the knees on the abdomen and then release. Repeat this movement several times. This action massages the colon and intestines and releases bubbles caught inside, thus the pain felt by your baby.

If your baby finds it hard to bend and relax the knees and legs, start by massaging each leg from the thigh to the foot. With both hands, hold your baby's thigh and do little pressure points by alternatively tightening and releasing your baby's leg from top (thigh) to bottom (ankle). Each action from you in the massage must be a firm but gentle and respectful touch.

o **Lactose Intolerant, Could It Be?**

This topic is linked to the one above 'Infant GERD' because most of the time a lactose intolerance can lead to gastroesophageal reflux. The symptoms are also similar and when your child is lactose intolerant or has a lactose overload (not the same cause) the major signs are spitting-up, non-stop crying, liquid/green explosive stools, nappy rash and agitated sleep.

Having said this, all babies will have these symptoms during the first weeks and months of life until about three months old, whether they are breastfed or formula-fed babies.

Most babies will have colic and some of the symptoms above, so it is necessary to wait until the intestines and digestive system become mature (about three months). Very young babies are often not yet producing enough of the lactase enzyme, which helps to digest lactose. If the symptoms are intense and that you notice that time doesn't seem to sooth your baby, it is time to seriously investigate.

When babies are breastfed, lactose intolerance can either come from a lactose imbalance or overload in your milk production or breastfeeding routine (I talk about this in the breastfeeding topic). Or, it can be that your child is really sensitive to lactose due to a lactase deficiency. But this is quite rare, and it is usually recommended to analyse and adjust your breastfeeding routine first.

Go back to the breastfeeding section and read again about milk supply, breastfeeding length and length between feeds. Whatever the case is, you can continue to breastfeed your child. Breastfeeding will always be the best thing for your baby and there is no such thing as your milk has a problem or is not good enough.

To stop breastfeeding or switch to a lactose-free formula milk is not the solution and it is only necessary in very rare cases after you have discussed this with your paediatrician and after doing some tests.

**If your baby is agitated before sleep**

Of course, a full body massage is the best, but you can just do a quick massage to relax your baby before sleep. You can either do a face massage or a foot massage, it's magic!

1.  Face massage:

First, start by massaging the forehead above the eyebrows. With your thumbs, start by placing them in the centre of the eyebrows (third eye) and swipe both thumbs at the same time towards the sides. Follow the eyebrow linage. Repeat three to five times.

Then starting in the same spot between the eyebrows, place your thumbs and swipe downwards on each side on the nose, continue to finish on the high cheekbones. Do it simultaneously with both thumbs. The movement must be firm but gentle and slow, it must flow. Repeat three to five times.

Place your thumbs under the nose, between the nose and the upper lip. With a slight pressure and with both thumbs, simultaneously slide to each side following the cheekbone lines. Your thumbs must be placed under the cheek bone line. Repeat three to five times.

Do the same movement starting with your thumbs in the middle of the chin and swipe to each side following the jaw line up to the ear lobes. Repeat three to five times.

To finish, place your thumbs on the tip on the chin and do little circles with your thumbs on the jawline slowly and gradually finish at the ear lobes.

2. Foot massage:

There are several foot massages but if there is one you must do, it's this very easy but effective one.

With both of your hands, take your baby's foot. With your right hand, place your thumb on the heel, the sole of your baby's foot and with your left hand place your thumb under the top bones (cushion that forms the top of the foot before the toes). One thumb after the other, starting with your right thumb swipe from the bottom of the heel towards the middle of the sole of the foot.

Again, press firmly but gently. Do the same movement with your left thumb swiping from under the top bone towards the toes. Repeat these movements alternatively five times. Finish by rolling each little toe with your index finger and thumb.

If you are interested in infant massage and would like to know all the techniques for the whole body, you can find a IAIM instructor in your area on their website www.iaim.net or buy the book *Shantala*, where every massage is illustrated with pictures.

I would like to share an extract from the book *Shantala*, which explains beautifully what your baby is experiencing and how he/she perceives the world: "It is essential to restore the balance. And to nourish the 'outside' with as much care as the 'inside'. To help babies get through the desert of the first months of life, so that they no longer feel the anguish of feeling isolated, lost."

"It is necessary to talk to their back, to talk to their skin, which is as thirsty and hungry as their tummy. Babies need milk, yes. But even more to be loved, and to receive caresses."

### o   The Importance to Cradle Your Baby

As I mentioned in the notion of bonding, especially the first weeks, your baby needs to be held, kept close against you or your partner. I use the word father a lot in the book but it also means the partner in the parental couple. We often think it has to be the mother who cradles, but the father can cradle his baby just as much. Your baby needs the warmth and the smell of the father as well. As you can't always do it all alone, ask your husband or partner to do the skin-to-skin cuddles and carry your baby in a scarf or in a physiological baby carrier.

I used the baby scarf carrier 'Je porte mon bébé' which is now called 'Love Radius'. They have a great collection of basic carrier scarves and physiological baby carriers. Their scarves are great to use because they are elastic. If you are an advanced baby scarf carrier, you can use any large cloth but if you are new to this technique, I strongly recommend you buy the right equipment.

If you want to be able to carry your baby around a lot during the first months, it's primordial that you are comfortable. It's also important that your baby is in the right physiological position, as close as possible to the foetal position your baby was in your tummy.

It may sound scary or complicated to use a scarf, but once you know the basic technique, it is very easy and quick to use. Love Radius have demonstration videos on their website www.love-radius.com. You can also search for tutorial videos posted by mums on YouTube.

To reassure your baby, connect and create a bond, there is a winner cocktail:

The right baby carrier + a good position + your warmth + your smell + movement = A HAPPY BABY!

Again, I say 'your', but your partner can do it too.

Now I am not saying this is magic and that your baby won't cry at all. But it will avoid a long list of unmet needs your baby expresses through his/her cries. And when your baby does cry, cradling is the best solution. When your baby gets older (after four months), the cries will become less frequent and less intense.

o   **How to Recognise Infant GERD**

For my first baby, I had never heard about Infant GERD (Gastroesophageal reflux disease). I discovered my baby was suffering from it when he was three months old. The main symptom of Infant GERD, which is a gastroesophageal reflux, is when your baby spits-up regularly during the day, even several hours after feeding, this followed by hours of crying.

Now this is quite a tricky one to diagnose by yourself because is it normal for babies to spit-up milk after feeding especially during the first weeks or months of life. It's also normal for babies to cry. The spitting-up is simply because the little valve in your baby's oesophagus is not mature and doesn't close properly until your baby is a couple of months old (until about three months).

There can be many reasons that explain these symptoms and usually it is because your baby has colic, needs to be cradled or is experiencing the evening cries.

However, in the case of Infant GERD, nothing seems to comfort nor calm your baby and you can sense despair in the cries. You can also notice arching of the back during and after the feeds. It's much more common for babies fed with formula milk to suffer from GERD. But it also happens with breastfed babies like in my case.

With hindsight, I know understand why my baby had Infant GERD despite being breastfed. As I explain in my breastfeeding tips, I had too much milk, making my baby get the wrong lactose balance which created colic and reflux. I now understand that the lactose imbalance in my milk may also have caused a lactose intolerance for my baby. This is not an irreversible situation, there are actions that can be taken and your baby will naturally outgrow this condition.

My advice is if you want to be sure your baby is suffering from Infant GERD, consult your paediatrician. My paediatrician easily confirmed the diagnosis by the redness and irritation in my baby's throat. If it's the case, there are several things that can be done to help your baby live this difficult period with more ease.

What can you do?

The actions I took on top of trying to regulate my milk production to minimise the lactose imbalance, was to make sure my baby was in a sitting position or straight position at least twenty minutes after breastfeeding. I would also raise my baby's mattress to make sure that he was never lying flat on his back.

For my second baby, I bought a 'Cocoon baby' by Red Castle. It helped me a great deal because it kept my baby in a physiological position close to the foetal position in the womb. This position helps minimise the symptoms of reflux and colic. It also reassures and reminds your baby of the comfortable and soothing environment of the womb.

I also noticed that it avoids your baby getting the flat skull problem, many babies suffer from due to inadequate sleeping positions.

I also gave medication after each breastfeed, called 'Gaviscon' for infants my paediatrician prescribed. I don't know if it really helped but the crying did last a bit less. I can remember feeling bad and having the impression I was intoxicating my small baby, but I was desperate for the suffering to stop.

You can also try lower-volume feedings, if you are using formula milk adding thickening agents (rice or quinoa cereal), changing for an anti-regurgitant formula, trying extensively hydrolysed or amino acid formulas. If you think your baby is lactose intolerant, change to a lactose-free formula. If you are breastfeeding, eliminate cow's milk and eggs from your diet to see if you notice any difference.

Usually, the lactose intolerance comes from the lactose imbalance in your milk and not from what you eat. But you can always try and see if there is a difference in your baby's reactions; if not, go back to eating what you like.

o **Anticipate and Sooth Teething**

This is also a tricky one to recognise when you are a new mum and even if you're not. Teething signs can sometimes be quite traitorous. Here are a few tips that can help you recognise the signs and anticipate the teething crisis.

Teething is when your baby's teeth start to come through their gum line.

Most babies start teething between four and seven months, but this is an average and there is no rule. Some babies are born with a tooth, some start teething at two months and others only at twelve months.

The teething signs depends on each baby. Some may show no sign at all and others all the signs, again there is no rule. All we want is to sooth your baby and make sure you and your baby suffer the least from these symptoms.

**The signs of teething:**

- Red, swollen gums
- Fever around the range of 37.5 C and 38.5 C (101 F) sometimes even 39 C but quite rare.
- A lot of drooling
- Runny nose
- Bad nappy rash
- Red cheeks (in the evening)
- Crying, fussy mood

- Greenish diarrhoea
- Bringing the hands to the mouth
- Rubbing cheeks or ears
- Disrupted sleep pattern

So, as I said, your baby won't get all the signs but generally a nice little cocktail of some of them. When we are busy mums, we are taken away in our routine and it is sometimes hard to stop five minutes, analyse the symptoms and make our diagnosis in order to decide which step to take next.

You may ask yourself: "Shall I consult my paediatrician, or have I noticed some changes in my baby that make me think he/she is teething?"

With my first baby, we lived in Paris and the first winter was literally hell. He started day-care in autumn at five and half months and I spent the winter with an ongoing sick baby. Having no experience, no help, it was impossible for me to recognise when he was teething. So as soon as he had a runny nose, fever, crying and difficult sleep, I would rush to the doctor who would tell me, either he is teething, either he has a virus that will eventually pass.

It is only with experience and a sense of taking a step back that I could observe my baby's symptoms and understand what was going on.

For example, if you notice your baby with red cheeks in the evening, a runny nose (but not to the extent of a huge cold), a lot of drooling and a bad nappy rash, you can be pretty sure your baby has a tooth or two making its way out. My baby during teething periods had such bad nappy rash, that it was almost to the extent of bleeding. It was awful!

**What can you do?**

There are several things you can do to anticipate, sooth and repair.

1.  Homeopathy

As soon as you notice the first signs of red cheeks, slight temperature in the evening, fussiness, and difficult sleep, it is a common sign of teething and can be treated with two homeopathic remedies: Belladonna 9 CH and Chamomilla 9 CH.

Some pharmaceuticals have prepared liquid solutions so it is easier to administrate to your baby, but I have a doubt on the efficiency. You can also ask your pharmacist to create a solution of both remedies with Weleda laboratories or you can simply buy the remedies and put two pills of each remedy in two drops of water. Let the pills completely dissolve and put the drops of water on your baby's tongue. Administrate a certain length of time away from any food, drink or medicine.

2.  Pain killers

If you notice your baby is fussy, crying, rubbing his cheeks or gums, that sleep is difficult that there is a runny nose or a nappy rash, give some paracetamol to relieve the pain. We know that paracetamol or ibuprofen isn't good for our health but when it is necessary, we shouldn't be against it. As long as there is no excessiveness in use or overdosage, it's fine.

As you know, a tooth pain can be unbearable, and we don't want to take the risk of leaving our child with such suffering.

3.   Bad nappy rash

My babies always had a bit of a red bottom now and then but when my first baby had a real crisis, it was already too late to avoid the suffering. Having no experience, I didn't know terrible nappy rashes could appear from nowhere and I didn't know it was because of teething. One evening, I picked-up my son from daycare and one of the ladies told me he had a bad rash.

I wasn't too worried but when I arrived at home, I was shocked. The same morning, he was fine and, in the evening, I couldn't touch him, he couldn't even sit-up without screaming. I gave him a quick bath, but his cries told me how awful it was. I put some cream and left his bottom free of any nappy/diaper or fabric, the contact was too painful.

**What can you do?**

What saved us with my baby was buying cotton pads at the pharmacy which are to be added in the nappy/diaper. I also got the repair cream 'Cicalfate +' from the French brand, Avène. I usually only use natural creams and products, but this cream is magic. I would apply the cream after a quick bath in the evening and add a cotton pad in the nappy.

By morning, just like that, the horrible nappy rash was almost gone! In one night, it usually disappears making it bearable for my baby the next day. What a relief! Whether the rash is bad or mild, never use wipes with perfume or alcohol, prefer a natural calcial lining ointment with non-bleached cotton. You can actually make your own calcial lining with organic olive oil and limewater.

**Homemade calcial lining ointment:**

In a glass bottle, ideally with a pump, fill-up half with olive oil and the other half with limewater. Shake well. You can add a couple of drops of organic calendula extract.

You can use coconut oil to hydrate your baby's skin and use the Cicalfate + cream only for bad rashes.

4.   Gum massage

When the gums are very soft and red, massaging with a soothing gum gel can help momentarily during a crisis. Ask your pharmacist advice for a baby gum massage gel. Apply on a clean finger and do circular movements on your baby's gums. It's not so much the gel that helps but the massage. If you don't have a soothing gum gel, simply do circular movements with your finger and massage as much as your baby will allow you to.

It will relieve some pain but also help the tooth come out sooner.

5.   Cradle and keep close

Teething is one of those periods where you don't sleep well and when the sleeping routine can get chaotic. Rather than try and fight this tiring period by trying to put your baby to sleep in her/his bed no matter what, just listen to your heart. Cradle, keep your baby close, don't fixate on the usual time schedule, your baby will eventually fall asleep.

Keep your baby close, either next to you in your bed or next to your bed. Feel free to try, the hard days won't last forever.

# Chapter Two
# Happy Mum

As you've read through my experiences, it's takes time to understand, learn and trust your capabilities. I felt so lonely with my first baby; lonely in the way that I desperately needed the support that I wasn't alone living these difficult situations with my newborn. I also needed the advice in tune with who I was. So, I questioned, sought for help, searched for values and truth that spoke to my heart and soul.

I have grown and acquired knowledge through life teachings, which as we all know can be very hard sometimes, but they are blessings in disguise. I am very grateful for all the people I have met on my path and who have guided me in very vulnerable situations. If I had had the opportunity to have access to these tips and tools at the time to guide me, it would have saved me a lot of time but mostly avoid a lot of worrying. And we know that worrying never does any good.

I now say this with a smile because I am so grateful to have lived these experiences.

All experiences in life come in polar opposites, from the terribly difficult, heart-breaking realities, to the wonderfully powerful understandings. This is the real notion of harmony, accepting the good and the bad for what it is, letting it be and keeping a happy balance within. Harmony is not perfection and a state of unwavering happiness. I am still learning to accept and keep this balance within. It takes time.

You probably heard this quote before but "Life doesn't happen to you, it happens for you."

In the next part of this book, there are seven fundamentals I would like to share with you. These fundamentals will help you understand, shift your perception of yourself and the world around you. It will help you access the power you have inside, the energy all human beings need in this life, but especially what a woman needs on the threshold of her new life as a mother.

- o Change your habits and understanding what a paradigm is.
- o Notion of love.
- o What other people think.
- o Shed the costume of guilt.
- o Learning how to respond.
- o Do things that make you happy.
- o Using tools for the mind and soul.

- o **Change Your Habits**

Now days, we are not used to listening to our intuition, we are not used to listening to the positive voice within us, we are usually judgmental and very harsh towards ourselves.

It is time mothers learn to love themselves and remove the guilt and pressure they may feel.

Today, even if things are slowly changing, we have this pressure of being the perfect mum, the perfect wife, the perfect businesswoman, the perfect everything.

Bob Proctor says in his last book *Change Your Paradigm, Change Your Life:* "We're being controlled by our outside world because we've been trained that way; we've been programmed to let the outside world control us."

It is time we train ourselves to take care of our inner world and let go of the image we have of ourselves or the label we were given.

Becoming a mum is already a life changing experience and it's not a matter of starting a psychotherapy here, on the contrary, it's very simple if you see it for what it is. It's a matter of awakening. When you give birth, in a way you are being reborn and entering a new chapter of your life: you are becoming a mother.

When you become a mummy, you are awakening a part of you that has always existed. I believe it helps us to learn how to act with more consciousness, to listen to ourselves, to listen to our baby. I mean really listen.

One of the ways to feel less influenced or controlled and thus, more in tune with ourselves is to change our habits. There is a term Bob Proctor used to talk about these habits that are ingrained in our cells and that I was completely unaware of, it's the notion of '**Paradigm**'.

Tara Brach, PhD and mindful meditation teacher, uses the word 'trance of the mind or thoughts', it's the same thing. I want to explain the notion of a paradigm because the principles behind the word are fundamental. I invite you to not focus on the complexity of the written word, but rather concentrate on understanding the notion and lessons behind the word. I invite you to follow me so we can understand together.

### What's a paradigm?

Bob Proctor taught me what a paradigm is and how to change it, in an online course in 2020. It sounded very technical, and it was the beginning of a real shift for me. Having read the books *The secret* and *The power* by Rhonda Byrne, I was familiar with many of the things he explained but I didn't quite get it at the time.

Let me say I got it intellectually, but not on the level I was supposed to perceive it to fully embody. But life has taught me that things arrive when we are ready, and I simply wasn't quite ready at the time. So, I continued my path learning differently with life experiences and special acquaintances (I call them guides). If you don't do your homework, life or the Universe will get you to do it one way or the other.

Being a big fan of Bob Proctor, I found out on his Instagram account that he had just published a new book called *Change Your Paradigm, Change Your Life.* He explains very simply what a paradigm is, he says: "A paradigm is a multitude of habits that are fixed in our subconscious mind." The subconscious mind is basically your habitual behaviour, things you do without thinking.

Most of our habits come from our childhood but they also come from our ancestors, in a way in runs in our blood. Bob Proctor says: "It's in our DNA."

The other habits and beliefs come from the outside world, from all the information circulating in the world and constantly feeding our conscious mind. Your conscious mind is the mind you think with and make decisions with.

A paradigm is formed with the way we were born in the world; it's the memory of difficult experiences we live in our childhood that create traumas whether big or small. It becomes with time, when we grow-up the little negative voice or the ego speech that can block us in life and keep us in the space of fear. This ego speech represents you as a person in the world, separate, and how you perceive the world through those eyes.

Most of the time we feel insecure, unloved and the ego speech or little voice can be something like "you are not good enough," "who do you think you are," "no one loves me" or "I am not doing things right."

Once we are aware of this, something happens, we awaken. We become aware of something we ignored. We go from ignorant to knowledgeable.

So, if we change this by implementing new habits in our subconscious mind and switching the negative talk to the positive whisper, it will become natural in our actions and thus, in the results in our life and around us. This applies to every area of one's life, but I thought it was essential to understand this notion in motherhood. There are so many things we need to handle as a mother, we need the solid grounds within us to support us.

For example, following the mind and soul tools I share in this book with repetition will do you good if you do it occasionally, but will do something magical if you do it with repetition, every day, on a longer period of time. It will change your old habits fixed in your subconscious mind (the things you do without thinking) and it will bring you real well-being and happiness inside.

First, you will just be aware of it and then you will use these nourishing tools spontaneously. You will be actively modifying your paradigm (habits). By changing your paradigm, you are learning to dimmer your ego and ultimately learning to feel truly good about yourself. What you think about yourself is so important.

By thinking everyday how worthy, capable, and beautiful you are, you will believe it. You will feel it, you will know it as truth.

As Bob says clearly in his book: "When you impress an idea over and over upon the subconscious, that idea must by law manifest through you."

Now, I wish to emphasise that only good thoughts will manifest through you because you truly wish for them with your heart. Negative thoughts or ideas are what you don't want, they will manifest through you too, but at least not as powerfully and fast as positive thoughts. You can see the negative thoughts as signals, here to warn you to take care of yourself. To shift your thoughts to a more positive vibrational mindset, even if it's just a little bit.

Being conscious of your thoughts and actions while pregnant, and during the first months of life of your newborn baby is essential. It's the foundation, the rich soil, it's the program, it's part of your future baby's paradigm. Again, this is not trying to be perfect; it's all about feeling, nurturing, giving love, transmitting the right habits and attributes.

Again, repetition is key here, so the tools I suggest further on must be implemented in your daily routine with repetition throughout the weeks to create new habits. Now I hear you, don't see this as a chore, it will bring you pleasure, true well-being and it will create balance in your everyday life. You are slowly changing your paradigm, your belief system for the good of your inner balance and self-love.

It will also prepare you for childbirth and create the right environment for your baby to be born in this world.

o **Notion of LOVE**

But what does LOVE really mean?

It's quite easy to start here, by mentioning the love of a mother for her child, to explain what love really is and how it feels. This love is the feeling you have when you hold your baby for the first time or when you bond with your child and truly get to know your baby (this can take several months). The love for your child is unique and pure.

It is that fondness, it is that sweet and yet strong and warm sensation you feel in your heart or that beautiful feeling you have in your stomach when your baby smiles at you.

But what does love mean in our world and how do we see it in others?

This very strong and powerful word used commonly in our daily conversations and in our habitual language loses its truthful signification. Love is usually assimilated to sentimental feelings, when you are romantically in love with someone or when you really enjoy something.

Dan Harris explains this in his podcast, *Ten Percent Happier, in part one of The Dalai Lama's guide to happiness*, after spending three weeks with his holiness in Dharamsala, India.

"Love is our evolutionary capacity to cooperate, communicate and connect. This allowed our species to thrive." So, the meaning of love I wish to open our hearts to is the loving kindness of just acknowledging our presence here and now. It's acknowledging the presence of others around us, seeing a person for who she or he is in that present moment.

Love is a powerful force and greatest energy we all have inside us and that we all share. It's the universal love where there is no gender, no age, no colour of skin. By looking in someone's eyes, you are saying "I see you," "I see your being." It's a very different feeling to sentimental or sexual love. When you do this 'seeing', something magical happens whether conscious or unconscious.

It may probably happen that the person feels very uncomfortable with the eye contact or on the contrary greets it with happiness and returns a smile. Try and stay there just for a fraction of a second. Did you feel that? This is love, this is what we all share.

We have restricted our hearts to love. By social conditioning, we have restricted our heart to love ourselves and therefore, love others and be able to give freely with no limitation.

But it's very important we understand that we must start loving ourselves unconditionally first, in order to be able to love others. As Rebecca Li, PhD and Chan Buddhist teacher, says: "To love ourselves, is accepting the good and the bad we have done, accepting our mistakes by facing the consequences, but we love ourselves anyway."

It's seeing ourselves for who we are now, acknowledging our own presence and holding space for the suffering we may have inside. When we can do this for ourselves, we can do it with others. In Buddhism, there is the saying: "We are all equal," we are all the same essence of light and love.

I experienced something extraordinary that is a perfect example. When I related my experience, some understood with a warm smile and others saw it with the walls and locked doors of separateness we live in. It happened in the subway last week while visiting my sister in Paris.

The vibes in the Parisian subway are heavy. I suppose it's more or less the same in every subway worldwide, but being very sensitive, I feel it a lot. I was sitting in the metro (subway) looking at people. Most people looked sad, empty, there was no sparkle in their eyes, that is, if I could even get a glimpse of them because no one looks at anyone. Everyone is locked in their protective field avoiding eye contact.

I am not judging here; I know how this feels as I have been there. I used to live in Paris for many years and I took the metro or bus to go to work every day. I had locked myself-up in protection, in defence of what could happen. I guess this is even more true when you are a pretty young woman.

While I was changing train and looking for an indication for the train line, a man with no ticket asked if he could pass the gates with me. He saw I hesitated for a second and reassured me that he would keep his distances. While I wasn't concerned about that, I accepted and asked him directions for the train I was looking for.

He really wanted to help me but he didn't know. Suddenly, someone turned around, looked at me and asked where I was going and politely showed me the way. He made sure I found the right track and the right train.

I thanked him genuinely for being so kind and helpful, doing so I looked into his eyes, like really in his eyes. He saw and I saw. This was not a romantic meeting or any feeling close to sentimental. It was just full of awareness in the moment. Acknowledging the person who was in front of me.

No matter the gender, colour of skin, age, looks, it was purely an acquaintance of two beings, of two souls.

Before my train left, he came back while I was reading *Light Is the New Black* from Rebecca Campbell. He told me: "I don't why, but I feel I must tell you that I am working on a project of finding ways for people to change the way they live and interact with others. We need more kindness and awareness, we can't continue to live this way, being selfish, separate, and living in fear. We must do it for us now, but especially for our children."

While we were looking into our eyes all this time, I felt tears in my eyes. I smiled and said: "I am on the same mission." I also take this as another sign from the Universe, signs I had been asking for.

We must open our hearts and allow ourselves to love freely. We must step out of fear, free ourselves from social conditioning, start showing kindness and love to lead the way for our children.

By putting attention on self-love daily, you activate a deep knowing. You are directly sending waves of love and trust to your whole being. If you're pregnant, not only is it powerful for yourself but it is pure nurturing love for your child. You are already raising your child, giving your baby the seeds.

To help you do this, I give you a self-love mantra to repeat daily and a guided meditation in Chapter Three, the Tools for the Mind and Soul. Don't let yourself get afraid by the word 'meditation', I stayed blocked there for a while. Meditation is nothing more than sitting with yourself for a moment and accessing this love, this universal energy. Meditation is taking care of yourself, of your inner world.

## o  **What Other People Think**

Another notion that may interfere with learning to love yourself as a mother, is worrying about what other people think. I used to worry so much about other people's opinions and what they would think of me. But all it does is drain your energy, add doubt to your capabilities and create anxiety. You must know that you are enough.

Healthy advice if you are asking for it is good but worrying what other people think of you will lead you nowhere.

Most of the time you have the answer, if you listen to that loving whisper you feel in your heart. It's always right, it's you. Deepak Chopra says it well: "The self is not in the realm of thought. It's in the gap between our thoughts. The cosmic psyche whispers to us softly in the gap between our thoughts. This is also what we call intuition." If you listen well, you will know when a 'yes' is a real 'yes' and a 'no', a true 'no'.

Trust your intuition, trust that gut feeling, it's never wrong. You will automatically seek for someone else's opinion to have the approval from an outside source but listen to you first.

This brings me to say, we worry about what other people think, but what do we think of ourselves?

Have you ever asked yourself, "What do I think of me?"

The most often, uncomfortable feelings come up. I know for me that it was "I am not enough," "I am not doing enough," and I felt guilt. Rather than fight against those feelings, push them away or shovel them back inside, feel your emotions, let them exist and then let them fade away.

Sometimes it takes time to be able to sit with our emotions, don't pressure yourself.

With time, you will naturally find the answers and the emotions will pass. You need to seek inside yourself for the soft, loving understanding and compassion.

The more you nurture your spirit, the more you feel love for yourself, the happier and more confident you will be. It will radiate from you like a powerful light, and give your child the gifts needed in life for a more loving and less separated world.

o   **Shed the Costume of Guilt**

How many times I have felt guilty as a mother? Don't we all?

Being a mother is the ground for guilt, feeling we are never doing enough or doing it right. And sadly, every day society puts us in situations of guilt and feeds us with information that is not true. It is time we show kindness to ourselves, it is time society shows kindness and compassion to mothers.

On my path to self-development and spirituality, I have so many times felt guilty for not being positive or not feeling good. There are different aspects to this feeling that once you are aware of, help shed the costume of guilt.

One of the aspects is coexistence of opposites. This notion is merely one of the basics of life and human nature, but Deepak Chopra in his book, *Creating Affluence,* explains it beautifully: "Joy and sorrow, pleasure and pain, up and down, hot and cold, here and there, light and darkness, birth and death. All experience is by contrast, and one would be meaningless without the other."

When we think about this in women's life, in motherhood, it removes a huge bag of guilt we've been carrying. You are allowed to feel down, it is normal to feel exhausted or to feel sorrow and pain. This does not make you a bad person or mean you are failing as a mother.

Rather, stop for a second, stop the thinking and observe with a kind eye what you are feeling. You are human, let the emotions be what they are and let it pass.

The other aspect is that this actually is a positive sign in disguise. When you are feeling down, sad, or angry, it is the perfect moment to work on yourself and grow.

Ask yourself: "Why am I feeling like this? Am I being too hard on myself? Have I held emotions inside that need to be expressed?" It is simply a sign that something needs to change or needs to be taken care of with a kind and loving eye. It is always an opportunity for you to expand and awaken.

## SHE

*Every day a mother does her best,*
*whether she is an organised or a messy type, calm or*
*shouter, tired or active,*
*everyday a mother does her very best.*
*She does it for her children, for her husband, for her family.*
*But what about her?*
*Most of the time this means she pulls strings inside, pushes*
*deep down emotions of unmet needs, misunderstandings,*
*judgment, or guilt.*
*She must ask herself "What do I think of me? How do I feel?*
*Do I love me?" When she goes and meets those emotions*
*inside,*
*when she is gentle and kind with herself, then she has the*
*tools to be her very best, in harmony with who she is and her*
*needs, to shed the costume of who SHE must be.*
*Charlotte Logan*

## o **Balance and Harmony**

As I explained before, emotions come in polar opposites. But there is also a general notion of opposites that helps understand the definition of harmony and balance in our lives.

Everything has an opposite, it can be light/dark, happy/sad, sunny/rainy, the Ying and the Yang. I am not a specialist in Chinese Ying and Yang philosophy, but it struck me one morning after my meditation. The Ying and the Yang represents the feminine and the masculine energy.

As we know there is an imbalance in our world between men and women. When we come out of patriarchism models and give more importance and space to women, a balance can arise between men and women, so between the Ying and the Yang energies. Perhaps only then, we will start to see what harmony really means in our world.

When there is an acceptance without judgment of the existence of polar opposites, when there is a balance between these opposites, then we understand the real notion of harmony. Harmony isn't everything is bright all the time, everything is happy, everything is perfect.

Harmony is accepting the good and the bad, the yes and the no, men and women and all opposing energies.

o **Learning to Respond**

We live in a world of action and reaction, in a world where everything goes fast all the time. We react to people, to situations, even to ourselves. While it is natural, we need to remember to think, maybe to slow down for a second in order to be able to respond.

It's hard to be a mother, it asks for a huge load of patience, discernment, compassion and poise. It's ever so normal to feel overwhelmed and explode sometimes. It asks for understanding, altruism, and support to manage certain situations.

Even the most daily insignificant situations, like when you are preparing your kids for school on a Monday morning and that they are constantly triggering you … and you explode. I am still working on it but the answer is to respond and not to react.

It is also true with any human being who may harm or upset us, we tend to react. The response is to take a step back inside, feel the emotion, be awake and see it. And know that you have the space inside, to think and respond rather than react.

Bob Proctor explains in his book: "In order to be able to respond instead of reacting, first of all, you have to become aware that you are reacting. You can react so fast. (…) If I'm responding, I take a look and think, 'I wonder why he said that?' You are allowed to not agree with what another person is saying but at least you can answer back with the right words and be less in the over emotional or screaming."

The right words will come out and you will feel more centred and legitimate. Basically, you do less harm to yourself first and consequently to others.

Tara Brach, a PhD, meditation teacher, psychologist and author, also explains it very well in her podcasts. One of her tools in order to learn to respond is:

1.  Look at the situation from your future self, the 'you' who knows. To make it easier to visualise and feel, imagine the 'you' at the end your life, the person who knows how each moment is precious and that it's your intention in the present that's truly important. When you feel this, you will start to feel more space inside, more power to dimmer the reactiveness.
2.  The second step is to make the U turn; it's to pause for a second, see that you are in a trance mode of anger or aggressiveness, to notice it, to take a step back, and to take the U turn. It's stopping for a second and asking yourself "what am I feeling?" and "why?" go and meet the anger or pain.

3.  Finally, find that love and compassion inside and direct it to yourself and fill the space.

Sometimes, it's not about the other person in front of us, and when it is, you will see the situation under another perspective and handle it differently. You will just be able to express how you feel to the other person with the right words. To respond, doesn't mean you become a wise Saint who accepts with a smile what you are being told or what you are enduring.

You are human and you feel, you are allowed to be upset or hurt. There is probably a very good reason to feel that way.

I insist on this point because now days we tend to emphasise a lot in self-development on how to be compassionate at all costs. Well, not at your cost. Being compassionate is seeing that the other person is suffering or overreacting, yes. But we are not forgiving without question what has been said or done.

What you can do, however, is quit the reaction mode, and relate to the other person or situation in a more true and grounded way. For example, "What she just told me, hurt me, I don't deserve this" and share from a genuine and loving space how this makes you feel. The other person may not like it, but you found the resources within you to respond rather than react. It takes a lot of courage to do this, and you can be proud of yourself.

o   **That Little Voice**

Who hasn't got that little voice within that judges you, that brings you down. I've always had it and the negative voice got louder with time. At the end of the day, if you recorded what that little voice was telling you, you would be shocked to hear how mean and demeaning it is. This is our ego talking, here to protect you and keep you in a dark but comfy little box.

It's also your paradigm, your habits coming in to make sure you don't change. Whenever, you start hearing that voice say "I hear you" and replace the negative thought about yourself with the opposite value or words.

For example, if you get up in the morning and look in the mirror and the little voice says: "F..., you look so awful" say "I hear you" and replace with "take care of yourself, I love you" and smile at yourself in the mirror. Put fresh water on your face, cleanse with a face gel and dry with a clean face towel.

Try and use the most natural cleansing product possible. It doesn't have to be organic but with less chemicals possible is best. Always hydrate your skin (most natural as possible too) and remember the eye area, it helps to prevent dark circles and wrinkles.

Go and take your cup of tea or coffee and get on with your day with the right vibrations of self-love and acceptance. This way, you will naturally give the right amount of energy to others with an open heart.

o   **Do Things That Make You Happy**

One of the best ways to feel good each day, is to do things that make you happy. It can be the smallest things like enjoying your cup of latte or tea, buying flowers for yourself, listening to the birds, walking to work on a sunny day or feeding the ducks at the park with your children. Whether you want to read a book, write, exercise, or watch an episode of your favourite series, do it!

Make your day enjoyable, life is too short to stay stuck in your everyday routine. Spice it up, listen to the wants you feel during the day and go to bed at night feeling happy and grateful.

Doing little things that make you feel good, that make you smile throughout the day and every day, will ultimately bring you a sense of happiness or joy. Deepak Chopra said: "Life naturally evolves in the direction of happiness. We must constantly ask ourselves if what we are doing is going to make us, and those around us, happy."

Doing things that make you happy, is also a way to live in the present moment. You are not in the mind of thoughts, you are connecting to the now, to your presence in the moment.

# Chapter Three
# Baby's Here

○ **Tools for the Mind and Soul**

We have been through the tips and tools during pregnancy and the tips for the first months with your newborn baby which are essential. It will help you feel reassured and more at ease in your day-to-day life with baby. But you also need the depth, the tools for the mind and soul to nourish yourself, feel more grounded and deal with what needs to be dealt with.

Whether it's in your inner world or in the outer one.

## Postnatal Mindful Meditation

There are many meditation techniques, and it took me until now to actually include meditation in my life habits. I always knew I needed to meditate, and I always knew that someday I would. I wasn't ready until one day I heard that little whisper telling me: "Charlotte, the answer is in meditation." Having said this, I felt a lot of pressure when thinking of implementing meditation in my life.

I grew-up as a child with Indian philosophy and spirituality taught by my parents which profoundly nourished me, but I had always found these particular teachings too strict. Thus, I had many preconceived ideas and I thought I had to follow a precise technique and path. It turns out that those specific teachings are simply not my path to take.

Today, I don't have a precise meditation technique and I don't follow one specific spiritual teacher. I was interested in 'Transcendental meditation' at one stage, but again I didn't want to get stuck in one technique. I may get there one day.

So, I started my journey searching, asking the Universe for guidance and receiving. I had never listened to podcasts before but it seemed like a good place to start. I found a podcast from New York, 'The Rubin Museum of Himalayan Art', with amazing spiritual teachers from all around the world.

Before the meditation, they sit down, talk about compassion, love, healing and harmony in relation with Buddhism art and spirituality. They taught me how to meditate and bring back my focus. They also taught me to feel and heal. One day, I had just finished one of their meditation sessions when I heard the host mention another podcast channel they had called 'Awaken'.

Whether I heard this for the first time in their podcasts or whether my conscious was ready for the next step, I immediately tuned in. Again, it is a place of pure knowledge and opening of the mind and heart. Writers, spiritual teachers, activists, wisdom bearers come and share their life experiences and what they learnt from it; it is amazing.

It also uninhibits as the speakers talk about their troubles and suffering and that it's normal. I felt I was not alone which is extremely important.

Seeking for inner peace and love is not seeking for wisdom perfectionism. My podcast journey lead me to finding Tara Brach, a PhD internationally known meditation teacher and author of bestselling books *Radical Acceptance* and *True Refuge.*

Her meditations guided me and still do today.

So, if you are new to meditation and would like to try, may I offer some guidance. In the following pages, there are some basic meditation techniques you can easily use every day for ten to twenty minutes.

Sit in a calm room or outdoors, make sure you will not be disturbed. You can create your special meditation space with some nice cushions, plants, or flowers, it's important to feel comfortable and safe. I love to light a white candle and an incense stick. I have several types of incenses, depending on the mood I am in, the period of the week, month, or season. If you don't like incense, a natural scented candle does the magic.

Cross your legs, hold your back straight but without effort, you can sit on a cushion on the floor, on your sofa, in a chair or on your bed. Pull your chin slightly in towards your neck. Close your eyes or keep your eyes open if you are more comfortable but keep a low gaze. Breathe in and out normally focusing on your breath.

Let your body sit without tension, loosen your jaw, drop your shoulders and breathe in and out without any conscious effort, feel your abdomen or torso follow the movement.

If meditation creates anxiety with the breathing, you can focus on the sounds around you rather than on your own breath. You can also use other techniques like a mandala necklace. Hold the mandala necklace in your hands and with your right hand, unroll the necklace one bead after the other until you get to the end. Start over again as many times as you need.

This will help you focus and not get overwhelmed by your emotions. Having said this, if your emotions need to come out, if you feel like crying, let it be. Don't restrain it, don't hold back.

Your thoughts will jump in, your mind will be turbulent, but it's ok and it's normal. Bring back your focus on your breath, on the sensations. After a while when you feel relaxed, imagine white, pure, beautiful light shining within. This light radiates from you like the sun on a hot summer day. Allow yourself to feel this light, feel the love, feel the magic of this moment happening in the now.

Be here with yourself, aware of your whole being, allowing yourself to be part of everything else. When I am there, I can actually feel the space around me, as if there were no more boundaries. I am in that field, in that higher frequency or universal energy.

Again, each time a thought comes to you, don't worry, just let it pass and come back to your breathing. When you want to finish your meditation session, slowly start moving your fingertips and toes. Become conscious of how your body feels, feel the sensations and when you are ready, open your eyes. And then just for a minute, let all that goodness settle, without analysing or thinking. Just let it all flow.

The benefits of meditation are numerous but it is known to rise your vibration, relax your entire being, reduce stress, help with sleep, bring clear focus, help reduce mood swings and feel that loving confidence from within. With repetition, it will infuse your day and follow you in your daily activities.

## Mantras

Self-love mantra

Close your eyes or if you prefer to keep them open, light a candle and look at the flame. Feel strong love for yourself and repeat:

I am worthy, I am true
I am pure essence of love
I am powerful
I am divine feminine energy, I am here now
I trust my inner voice, I trust in myself
I trust in my capabilities, I belong
I am ME
I am HOME

You can say it over and over again, as much as you need, to truly feel it in your heart. To feel deep inside the acceptance and the trust. Doing this is easy, fast and efficient. It's like a mini meditation you can do anywhere. Whenever, you feel overwhelmed, doubting yourself or feeling very negative, stop, take a deep breath, close your eyes and repeat the mantra.

Personal mantra

Why don't you try creating your own personal mantra?

After a meditation session or when you feel in tune with yourself, ask yourself what are your qualities, what are you known for, who are you when you listen to the loving voice?

My personal mantra would be something like this:

I am loving

I am strong

I am authentic

I am a good listener, I am a healer

I am a teacher, I am caring

I am true, I am LOVE

## Perineum re-education

Before you can start exercising again, you must restore the strength of your perineum (pelvic floor muscle). The rehabilitation of the perineum can start usually two to three months after birth. It's an effective physiotherapy treatment with contraction exercises in the local pelvis area supervised by a midwife or specialised practitioner.

Once you have finished your sessions, your midwife will give you the green light to start exercising. It's primordial to re-educate your perineum muscle to avoid incontinence or even an organ descent. You may feel you don't need it or that it's not necessary, but I can tell you, you don't want to have to deal with these real physiological problems that are very hard to cure once they exist.

Having said this, the only exercise you can allow yourself to do before the perineal rehabilitation (even right after birth) is postnatal yoga exercises. Postnatal exercises actually protect your pelvic floor muscles and help your uterus go back to its original size. While this will happen naturally after the following weeks of giving birth, the exercises accelerate the process and help your uterus finds its original size and place.

Your pelvic floor has been through a lot of strain and this can be even more true depending on the type of birth you had.

I went to my yoga teacher, Sophie Colombié; newborns were welcome so I went there with my baby, where I could breastfeed if needed.

Sometimes, I couldn't attend the whole class because my baby wasn't too happy about it, but taking this time for me, meeting other mums and listening to Sophie; bathed me in an accepting atmosphere where I could belong. These were precious and indispensable moments.

I have prepared a little program of five postures and breathing techniques you can do alone at home. It's a mixture of the postures I preferred, that really helped me and the practices Sophie Colombié, my prenatal/postnatal yoga teacher, encouraged us to do at home. Doing this every day or even several times a day is efficient enough to help the recovery of your uterus and protection of your perineum. You will need a yoga mat and a large cushion.

Repeat the following exercises up to three or five times in a row. If you had a caesarean, you must wait at least two weeks for the following exercises, or more depending on how your scar has healed.

## Perineal exhale lying down

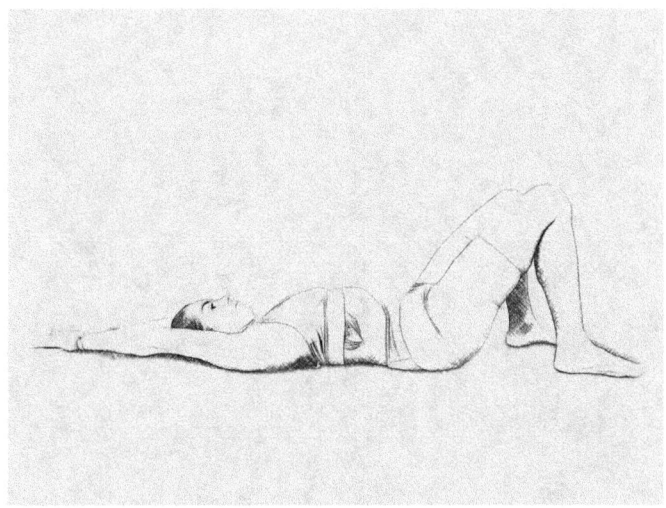

Lie-down on your yoga or gym mat and bend your knees. Breathe-in while bringing your hands together and hook your index fingers together. While you exhale, bring your arms above your head, arms straight and strong as if your wanted to push a wall behind you. Come back while inhaling, start again and this time while you exhale bring your arms above your head, push with your feet on the floor.

This will retrovert your pelvis (flatten your lower back) and mechanically pull-up your perineum. You will feel your tummy sinking in and your thorax opening. Your perineum needs gentle awakening and protection after what you have been through. Stay like this for fifteen seconds then come back while inhaling. Breathe normally.

## Perineal exhale and block sitting up

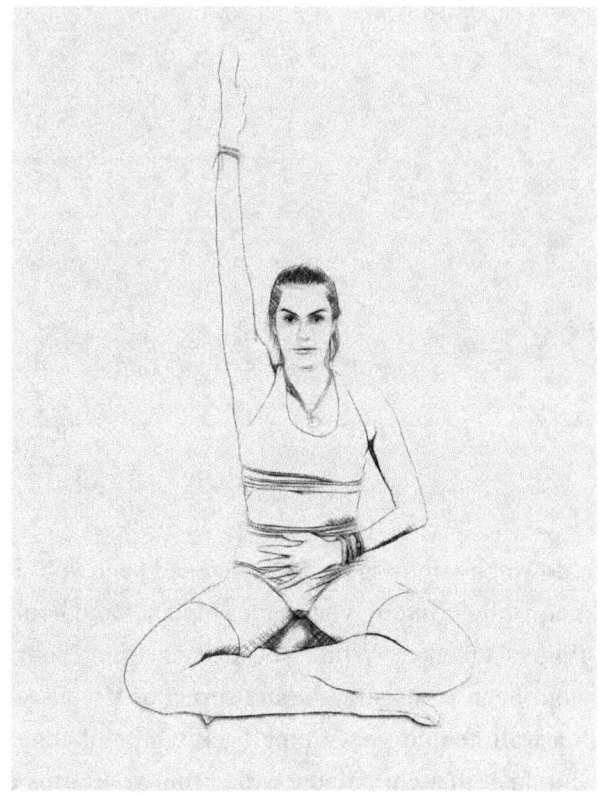

This exercise is quite technical, don't worry if you don't get it immediately. I found it very hard to grasp the first time, you will understand the more you do it.

Being very technical it is thus very efficient, it strengthens and brings your perineum back-up. Your perineum has been carrying a baby for nine months, it's a muscle that has been tremendously solicitated and stretched. This exercise also accelerates the process of your uterus getting back to its normal size. It will energise this area of your body and protect your organs.

Sit on a yoga mat or on a carpet. You can also sit on a cushion or in your sofa if you feel more comfortable. Sit crossed-legged or with your feet on the floor as long as your back is straight in a comfy way. Put one hand on your belly and the other in the air or on your solar plexus.

Start by feeling your breath. Take a deep breath, then breathe out and empty all the air you have. Your belly and chest should feel empty. Now the next step is to block the back of your throat and nostrils and pretend to breath in again, we want to use the action here but without taking in any air. It is important you don't take a real breath and block properly.

This action will suck in the remaining air left in your lungs, your chest will get bigger as if you were taking a real deep breath. Your belly however is being pull-in powerfully and is completely pulled back towards your spine. Your diaphragm is being sucked-up, contracting and by this action pulling your perineum up as well. This an amazing perineum re-education method.

With this technique, your uterus is contracting and being put back to its original place and size.

## Downward facing dog (Adho Mukha Svanasana)

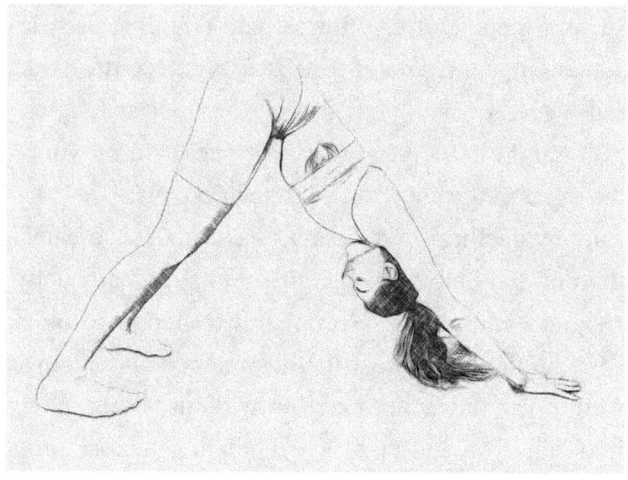

Stand-up your legs slightly larger than your hips. Bend down to form a bridge face facing down. Put your hands flat on the floor with your fingers open like a star. Your heels don't have to touch the floor, if you can't, it's fine, leave some space. Now push on your hands, arms straight and dynamic as if you wanted to push the top of your bottom in the air and backwards.

Let your head drop and breathe. Your legs are straight and dynamic. Stay like this for fifteen seconds. Then come-up slowly, unrolling your spine from the bottom right up to your head.

## Upward forward fold wall (Ardha Uttasana wall)

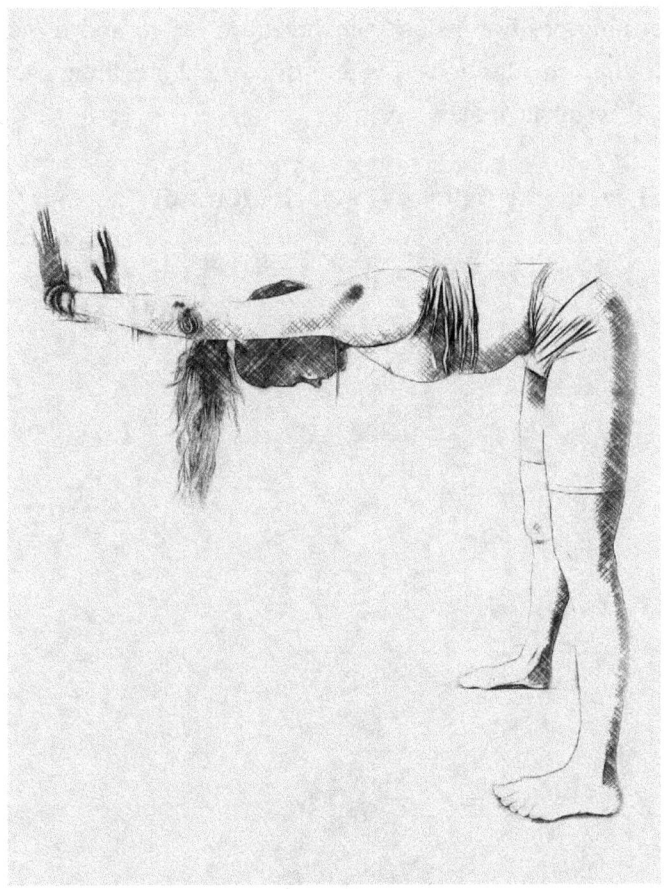

Stand legs straight in front of a wall, bend over 90° putting your hands flat on the wall, fingers open like a star. Make sure your arms are straight and strong. Adjust the distance between the wall if needed. Take a deep breath and when you exhale push the wall with your hands keeping your legs straight. Make sure your back is straight and not sagging.

To help you, bring your belly towards the back of your spine and your tail bone slightly towards you. Stay in this stretching position using your breath to let go and feel the sensations in your body. Do four or five full breathing cycles like this (inhale/exhale).

**Legs up the wall pose (Viparita Karani)**

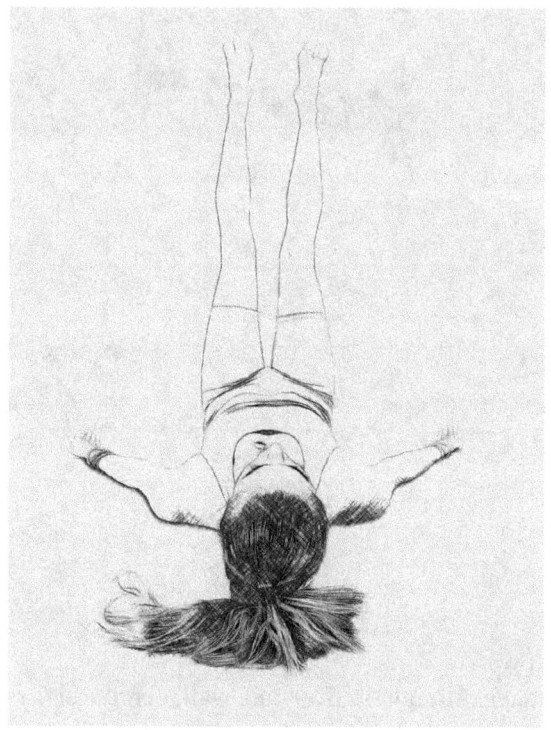

You will need a fat cushion, a mat and a wall. Sometimes your best friends are not who you expect. ☺

Put your mat against the wall and place the cushion on top against the wall too. In the Iyengar yoga classes I attend, we have ropes to help us bring our legs in the air, at home we do with what we have. Try sitting on the cushion sideways, thigh against the wall and then slide to bring your legs in the air against the wall. Your bottom must be as close as possible to the wall, on the cushion and your legs straight.

This is a wonderful way to relax your abdomen and activate your blood circulation.

## Postnatal stretching postures and toning after baby

As you know, don't try any exercises especially if you are not supervised before **three months postpartum** and you must do your perineal recovery with a practitioner or midwife first.

You only need three yoga postures and a couple of toning exercises you can repeat two to three times every morning, before your shower or when you have a fifteen-minute break. The benefits are amazing, you will feel energised, more centred from within, and you will strengthen your core muscles without damaging your pelvic floor. Remember to breathe when you do the postures and take the time to feel the sensations in your body during each posture.

I am giving a specific program that worked for me but feel free to adapt or change one or two exercises to others you find or prefer. The most important is that you stick to it and make it a habit, so make it enjoyable!

For the exercises, you will need a yoga mat and a long stick (broom stick without the head).

## Plank

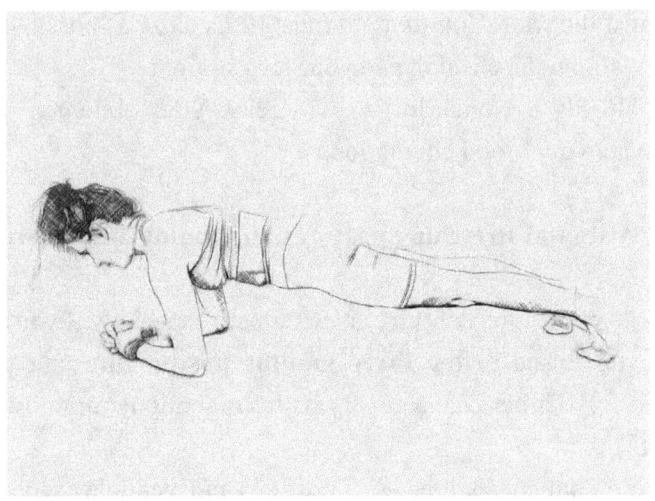

This is a famous one and I'm not teaching you anything here, it's just a reminder to put it in your exercise routine. You will need a yoga mat.

You can either do it with your arms straight or your arms folded 90° on your forearms and elbows.

The most important notion in this exercise is to make sure your back is straight and your neck and head aligned with your back. The bottom of your back mustn't sag. Make sure you use all your muscles, arms, back, bottom, tummy and legs. If you feel you are putting more effort on one part of your body, try and feel it and rebalance the effort you are putting in your muscles.

Make sure your tummy is pulled towards your spine. Start staying thirty seconds like this until you can stay for sixty to seventy seconds.

## Lateral Broom stick slides

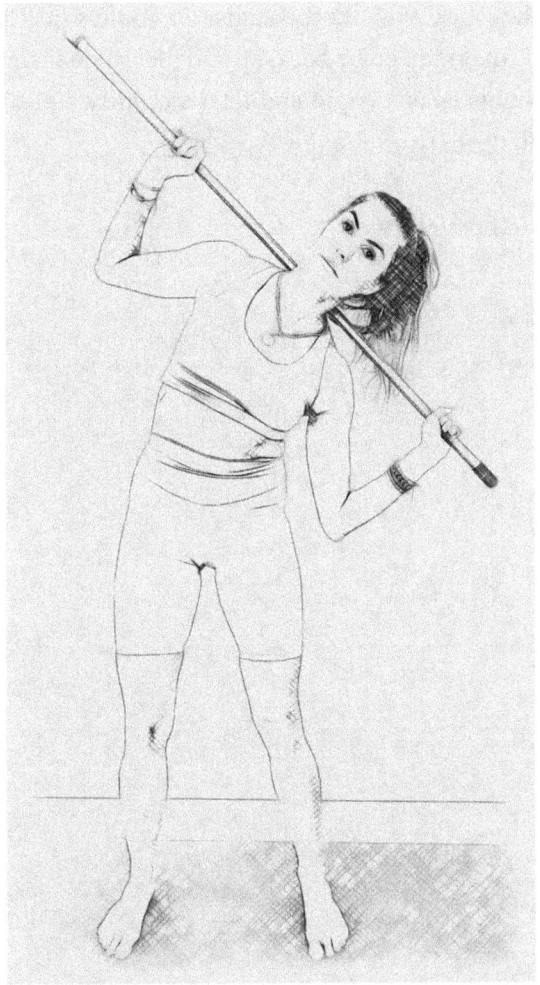

This exercise and the next one is great to tone and get your waist back! Use a long stick or a broomstick without the heat. It's easier to do the exercise in front of a mirror so you can see if you are doing the slides correctly.

Stand-up and put your legs hip width, slightly bend your knees. Place the stick behind your neck on your shoulders, hold the stick with both hands on each side. Now slide towards the right, come back-up and then slide towards to left. This counts as one (right and left), do thirty side slides until you can do sixty after a few weeks.

**Broom stick twist**

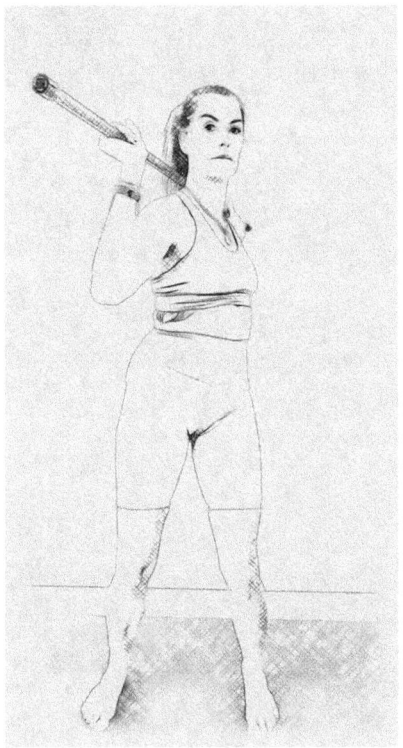

You start in the same position as in the previous exercise, but this time turn towards the right and then the left. This counts as one (right and left). Do thirty twists until you can do sixty after a few weeks. Important, make sure your hips stay straight, facing the mirror or wall. They shouldn't turn when you go right and left, only your waist and the top of your body moves.

**Bottom lift**

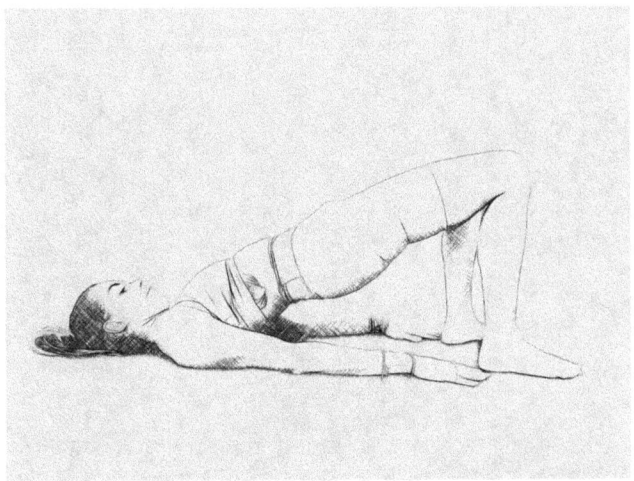

You will need a mat for this exercise.

Lie down on your back, bend your knees. Place your arms straight on each side of your body on the floor, palms facing downwards. Now bring-up your bottom towards the ceiling, and bring back down. Repeat thirty times. When you arrive to the thirtieth push-up, keep your bottom in the air and contract your butt muscles for twelve seconds. Then slowly unroll your spine and relax.

## Feet in the air abs

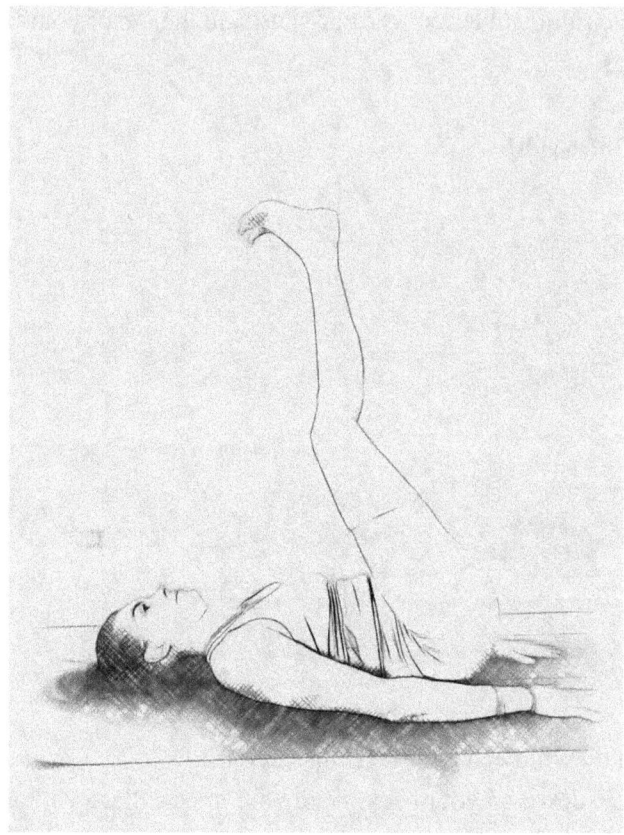

You will need a mat.

Lie down on the mat, place your hands out on each side of your body, palms facing downwards. Bring your legs up in the air bending your knees slightly. Keep your legs and feet joined together. Now with the strength of your abs and the aid (a little) of your hands lift-up your bottom, your whole bottom must lift-up from the ground. Then come back down, repeat twenty times.

## First month of sleep

Now this may sound 'cliché' but sleep is so important for a new mother. Now I know how easy it is to say but very hard to do. I am mainly talking about the first month after birth with your newborn baby. Later it may be more difficult with work or having other children to look after. If you can squeeze in a nap now, it's always extremely beneficial.

In many cultures during the first month, mothers are taken care of like queens (that we are). They stay in bed, sleep when they need to, some use bandage techniques around the pelvis and stomach to help the uterus and organs get back into place. Their families cook for them, bring them meals in bed and tend to the baby if she is resting.

In the West, we don't have this support and we are not used to asking for help. In our individualist society, we are used to taking care of things ourselves and putting our interest or health after our children.

Of course, our baby is amazing and needs all our attention but mummy you have grown, carried and given birth to a human being, you have accomplished something extraordinary. Rest as much as you can the first month and ask for help from your family, partner or friends. I did not ask for enough help, and with time it builds up inside.

## Power foods

The main power foods you may already know are *garlic, blueberries, broccoli, quinoa, oats, eggs, spinach, kale, almonds, goji berries, spirulina and chia seeds*. There is also salmon but I'm vegetarian.

After you give birth, your body needs a lot of healthy nutrients to recover as well and as fast as possible to be able to cope with the long interrupted nights. If you are breastfeeding, you will need the energy and it will help the production of your milk and maintain a good supply. Important notion it's about you here, not your baby or others.

It's about what you have been through (birth), the transformative state your body is going through (huge hormone change and physical readaptation) and the lack of sleep. It's about taking care of you, so now is not the time to start new smart recipes or elaborate ways of cooking, this would not be taking care of yourself but just adding more work and putting pressure on yourself.

On the contrary, you can eat healthy just by taking interest in what is good for you in this specific moment of your life. Simple interest in healthy foods or power foods and very simple cooking is enough. Listen to your needs and cravings. Just know that any over craving or over eating of industrial, transformed foods or sweets will affect your energy and health real time.

You preciously need this energy for you and your baby. The positive outcome will also be that you will get used to this new way of eating and you will take pleasure in it. Eating less meat and more natural and simple foods will impact many areas of your life and life around you. When your baby is a bit older, you will be able to test new recipes and also enjoy making healthy and fresh mashes for your baby.

For my second daughter, I was very implicated in healthy eating and power foods. I used to make power bowls every morning before my fifteen-minute postnatal workout. There are many power bowl recipes on internet and blogs. I would use plant-based milk, plant-based protein powder, bananas, blueberries, spirulina powder and I would decorate with coconut or cocoa nibs, chia seeds or fresh cut fruit.

Basically, just test and try out some mixtures and have fun. Most of my bowls looked very professional but I was just a beginner having fun!

**Here is one of the recipes I used most:**

- One banana
- Small handful of blueberries
- One scoop of vanilla plant-based protein powder (organic and health stores)
- 'Organic burst' Açai berry powder or Chlorella (Organic burst is a UK based company searching the globe for power foods in an ethical and sustainable way)
- Half a cup of oat milk (adjust to your taste)

A quick idea for rushed mornings is to prepare a chia pudding in the evening before going to bed. It literally takes five minutes. Make individual servings in little glass jars. I used to make some for my son who loved it! You can add cocoa powder or red berries to make it fun and tasty.

**Recipe**: 3.5 tablespoons of chia seeds, 1 small jar of oat or dairy milk and a bit of agave syrup to sweeten. Stir well three times, cover the jar and put in the fridge. In the morning, add fresh fruit or just eat as it is. It's delicious, full of fibre, omega-3s and a good level of protein.

### Boost your immune system

With the short nights and changing seasons, your body needs a boost to keep-up with your new busy routine and avoid catching all the viruses hanging around. Your baby may have started day-care and she/he will bring lots of microbes back home.

If you're still breastfeeding, ask for an adapted multivitamin complex in your local pharmacy or health shop. If you are not breastfeeding, you can do a complex of magnesium, vitamin C, vitamin D, vitamin Bs (especially B12 that usually women miss more than men because we usually eat less meat), zinc and selenium. You may also need some iron too, but it is best to do a blood test first to check your levels of iron to know what dosage you need.

I highly recommend doing a cure of probiotics for three months, especially during the autumn and winter seasons if you want to avoid those long colds or coughs.

The microbiota of your intestines and colon when unbalanced and weakened will affect your immune system and immunity to viruses.

### Baths with essential oils

*What you must know before using essential oils:*
While most essential oils are not recommended during pregnancy, there a couple you can use safely after the first trimester. You must always put your essential oils in a special neutral bath oil before putting into the water, some essential oils burn and can create skin irritations. You can put five

drops of each essential oil if you mix three types together or twenty drops of one type in your warm bath.

Attention! No burning hot baths. I know I love my baths to almost burn me, but it's very dangerous for you and your baby.

If you are postpartum, you can have your first bath after a month.

- **Geranium rosat**: Put twenty drops in your bath solution and pour into your running warm bath. Geranium rosat has a wonderful smell and helps with rheumatic pains, heavy legs and haemorrhoids. My advice is to not use this one if you still have your sickness problems. The smell being quite strong and powerful could put you off very quickly.
- **Fine lavender**: Put twenty drops in your bath solution and pour into your running warm bath. This essential oil is one of the most tolerated by all. It is wonderful for nervosity, insomnia, stress, irritability and sore muscles.
- **Mandarin**: Put twenty drops in your bath solution and pour into your running warm bath. This essential has such a lovely perfume, zesty and fresh. It is good for stress, nervosity and anxiety.
- **Sweet Orange**: Put twenty drops in your bath solution and pour into your running warm bath. It's similar to Mandarin but the perfume is slightly different and this essential oil helps for heart palpitations. I had quite strong palpitations during my third pregnancy, and it calms a lot.

- **Scots pine**: Put twenty drops in your bath solution and pour into your running warm bath. This one is just great for general fatigue and relaxes wonderfully.
- **Ravintsara**: The must have! It's my magical potion. It's mostly a powerful anti-viral but to me it's magic for just about everything. Fatigue, insomnia, nervosity, low mood. A few drops and your will feel regenerated.
- **Therepentine**: Put twenty drops in your bath solution and pour into your running warm bath. I have never used this one, but it is great if you are subject to lumbago or sciatic pains which we frequently have during the last trimester of pregnancy.
- **Vetiver**: Put twenty drops in your bath solution and pour into your running warm bath. Vetiver is perfect for circulation problems which we also have during the last trimester. It's also good for stress or a down mood.

  You can also make your own mixture of two or three essential oils. Just make sure you put twenty drops in total.

## Artificial but essential

Hairdresser, manicure/pedicure, hair removal etc. this may sound artificial or superficial, but it is essential to feel pretty, to feel feminine, and to feel fresh again! You are a mother, but you are overall a woman, a beautiful luminous being that needs to take care of her genuine beauty. No one ever complained after being pampered.

The notion of taking care of our self in motherhood is very important, and doing things for you, that make you feel good is fundamental. Like Beyoncé says in one of her latest songs "I am my own foundation;" this foundation makes everything else possible. The other day, I went to a manicure spa with one of my best friends who has a young baby.

While we were being looked after with our feet in a warm bubbly jacuzzi for the feet, we looked at each other and said: "Gosh this is really what I needed, time for me and to talk to a good friend." Moments like these are important and will help you stay balanced within.

## Massage

Book yourself a postpartum massage, the practitioners are trained to do specific massages that your body needs to recuperate, find the balance and energy for the coming months with your newborn baby. If you can't find someone specific, an essential oil massage is just as good and it can be very potent for creating a hormonal balance and improving your mood (this is linked).

The benefits from massages are numerous like reducing pain, reducing swelling, improve milk production, hormone regulation (helps avoid the hormonal roller coaster), reduce anxiety and depression and helps you with your sleep.

If you've had a caesarean or if you had blood clots, please ask your doctor advice before booking a massage.

## Babystroller gym classes

I never tried as I am into yoga but I have heard so much good about these classes. It is very hard as a young mum with your newborn to find the time for you, to start taking care of your body again. Babystroller gym classes take place in pretty green parks, you get to meet other mums and your baby gets to have a stroll.

It is so important to surround yourself with nature to rejuvenate and to meet other mums so you can connect. You will feel less alone, and you can exchange your tips or worries in a safe group.

## Music classes with baby

I did baby music classes with my third child in Lisbon. It took place in one of the most beautiful parks of Lisbon, Guerra Junqueiro Garden, also known as Jardim da Estrela. There are exotic ancient trees and a variety of beautiful birds. Just sitting there on the grass with my little girl in the morning was already a treat for my soul and for my general wellbeing.

But then, we had this amazing music teacher and musician Helena from 'Music room' school in Lisbon, who would come with her instruments and theme for the day. With a group of other parents and babies from all nationalities, we would chant, play instruments, listen to Helena singing and we would all dance together. We would let the babies interact with each other and respond to the music and sounds. Truly a magical moment to share with your child.

# Chapter Four
# Seeds for the Future

o   **Let's Change Things Together**

## Mother

*I am not a feminist*
*I am not a radical*
*I am a woman who has witnessed*
*unfair, hard, humiliating words,*
*attitudes or acts that can damage your soul.*
*It's a fact, not a march against anyone*
*or anything. It just is.*
*The truth is and will always be,*
*that women are strong, courageous, raw, loving*
*and overall indispensable to the future of this planet.*
*Behind every man, organisation, creation, or government,*
*a woman or women are working their magic.*
*Secretly, patiently behind the scenes*
*without waiting for anything in return.*
*Isn't that the key to success everyone is preaching about?*
*No fight can change the problems in our world, only love.*
*One day women who are the very prime essence of love,*
*will change things.*
*They already are.*

*Charlotte Logan*

## Medical and obstetrical violence

You probably noticed throughout my book that some of my experiences, whether it was for the early loss of my first baby or for my other childbirths, some things are just wrong. I voluntarily didn't make any comments because I don't have any judgment regarding the situations or the people who acted or managed in a certain way but there is a real problem.

Funny how when you are writing, flashes of a memory come-up and you realise that there is a wound there that has not yet been healed. I remember one of the first osculation I had in a clinic for my first baby (I lost) was extremely painful and humiliating. The doctor was a man clearly at the end of his career. He didn't even look at me and acted mechanically without any consideration.

I was a young pregnant woman with an unplanned baby so maybe I had less value to him? That's certainly the way he made me feel. The osculation in itself was worse, he was brutal, he pressed on my cervix so hard and roughly, I thought he was trying to interrupt my pregnancy.

He got up, threw his glove in the bin, and still without looking at me, said, "All is good." I left the hospital feeling violated, vulnerable and physically hurt.

When I went to see my general doctor for my first breast engorgement, early mastitis symptoms, rather than giving me a specific antibiotic treatment and sending me to my midwife for the practical tools, he tells me to do a cervix fluid sampling to be sure there is no infection. Just a reminder, I had given birth three months earlier, needless to say that the idea of having someone look at my private parts again and fiddle with my cervix was torture.

Meanwhile, I contacted my midwife who gave the steps to handle the mastitis. For the cervix sampling, my doctor told me: "I would change laboratory this time because sometimes laboratories get used to you and don't do their work as well." What a strange and weird thing to say to a patient who just gave birth and who is lost and exhausted.

So, against my intuition telling me to not bother changing, after all I felt safe in the lab I knew and it was next to my house, I searched for another laboratory.

I passed by a laboratory while taking a walk with my baby in the buggy. It was urgent and it wasn't too far from home. Again my intuition was trying to get my attention. I didn't feel good about this place at all; the location, the window, the people who greeted me. Nothing felt right. However, with my prescription in hand, I went in.

I was anxious because I was scared my baby would wake-up and start screaming. This was a rough time for me, my baby would cry a lot and I apprehended the cries. The laboratory owner and doctor told me he would do the sampling. I didn't like his vibes either and before he actually did anything, he was already assuming I had an infection or some kind of disease that only he could detect because he analyses within minutes rather waiting an hour like other labs.

Again, what a violent and cruel way to treat a young mother who just a few months away survived a tsunami, who is exhausted with the lack of sleep, who is probably very lonely at home and coping with the overwhelming waves of the rebalancing of her hormones.

The sampling itself was a horrible experience. The doctor was there with two assistants, all three of them looking at me with my legs wide open. My baby started to cry as if he was warning me. The sensation of the stick rubbing my cervix after a fairly recent birth was very unpleasant and intrusive. The Doctor took an awful amount of time and insisted with his examination stick.

My cervix started to bleed and he immediately said that this was bad news and that my uterus probably had an infection and that I could become sterile for life. Needn't he knew from his lack of knowledge that I had a **cervical ectropion**.

*Cervical ectropion means that the cells inside your cervix are visible outside of your cervix. Cervical ectropion isn't a concerning condition.* It's perfectly normal to bleed and I had always had a fragile cervix with contact. My baby was screaming like hell so the doctor tells me he will quickly analyse the sample and give me the results. I leave the lab feeling violated both physically and emotionally.

Two days later after the week-end, I receive an alarming call from the lab and from my doctor telling me I had to quickly treat a sexually transmitted disease. I tell my doctor how shocked I am and that there must be a mistake. I felt the heavy weight of judgment and lack of compassion when he tells me to consult my gynaecologist for this matter.

My gynaecologist, although being a woman, didn't greet me nor consider me better. With a cold and judging look and attitude told me, it was severe and that I had to be treated quickly as well as my husband. She also told me that I ought to think twice about my husband's fidelity. Now I understand that professionals act with facts, but I was in such shock for what I was being told, but mostly by humankind.

How can a young woman who just gave birth and who is vulnerable be treated this way without any warmth or consideration. Knowing my husband and our strong trusting relationship, the accusations didn't hold ground. I knew deep down this was a huge mistake.

I immediately called my midwife who was also shocked by what I was telling her. She told me to do another sampling to double check the results. The very same day, I went to my normal lab next door. While having the sampling done, I tell the woman why I was doing these tests.

She reassured me by saying that just by the look of my fluids and cervix that I was perfectly healthy. And as I had always known deep inside, the results came out clean.

I felt such anger and injustice. I called my gynaecologist to tell her how outrageous this whole experience was which simply started with a misdiagnosis of an early mastitis!

I sent an email to my general doctor telling him I wanted to denounce the owner of the lab to the medical order. He refused and said these things can happen.

I changed doctor and gynaecologist the very same day and showed the second results to the lab owner and left him standing there with confusion.

A few months later, when I consulted a new gynaecologist, I told her my story. With a comforting assurance, she told me to go to a lab specialised in biology for the third and last sampling test. The results came out clean and the last remains of self-doubt disappeared which allowed full healing inside.

There is clearly a lack of empathy, compassion, support and means. For some, it may be a trait of their personality, for others a protective shield or others just plain ignorance. This said, situations like this simply should not exist, you are allowed to say no. You are allowed to say stop. Listen to your intuition, I didn't listen to mine enough in those days. Listen to your voice within, your voice must be heard and we can change things together.

**Organising adjustments**

It's not a matter of insurmountable change, change comes with small adjustments, it's a matter of balance.

Change doesn't mean it has to be drastic, but rather adjusting the way things are handled in hospitals, what doctors, nurses and midwives learn at school and how mothers learn about their bodies, connect with themselves, and trust their inner strength.

The 'adjustments' to bring change are basically knowledge and training in several fields. When combined together, powerful evolution can take place in the collective.

If the efforts are made in the three following areas, real change and harmony will arise.

- **Medical training: Adapt theory learnt at school for doctors, nurses, and midwives.**

I am extremely grateful for all professionals in the medical field who devote their lives and energy by helping others. It is a noble and courageous path. The medical teams are here to save lives, avoid any unnecessary risks or danger and make sure mother and child are healthy. The way things are today, they do not have the luxury of time and means to get involved with each family, it is just not feasible.

And for obvious reasons, they do not get involved emotionally to protect themselves, this becomes natural with time. The automatism is to keep things very technical, efficient and unpersonal. It is a necessity and doctors, nurses, and midwifes should learn at school to have a protective 'airlock'. However, where the huge lack of training operates is in the learning of how to handle their patients' emotions.

All medical staff need to know how to handle traumatising experiences like death of newborns at birth, or how to accompany new parents in a very specific situation where emotional needs are big. They need to learn about personal growth and the impact their attitude has on women in very vulnerable situations. When you work with human beings and their emotions, the first thing to learn is compassion, kindness and intuitive intelligence.

- **Hospitals: Adjust protocols and organisation within the hospitals, choices given to mothers**

It's adjusting the hospital birth protocols by a less sterilised environment, removing the systematical stirrups, the early IV fluids, the heavy loaded epidurals, the systematic and elective c-sections, and the other impetuous things that can be delayed or removed. We go to the hospital or maternity to give birth, to give life not to have an operation.

But rather we should allow mothers to walk around, stretch and breathe in the birth room, install IV fluids in the last phase of childbirth if needed, suggest epidurals that relieve pain during the long process of labour but gently disappear while giving birth to fully follow the natural process of childbirth, create intimate environments in the birth rooms.

The medical assistance has gone too far and while it may make things easier for the doctors and hospital management, it creates an environment of fear, anxiety and rigidity. In this environment, it is almost impossible for any woman to give birth with self-confidence and in connection with her capabilities.

Adjustments in the way things are managed don't necessarily lead to less efficiency or more costs for the medical field. It's a matter of collaboration with all parties (staff, infrastructure and mothers) to have efficiency and satisfaction in a more conscious and aware way. And on top of this, new services can be offered to mothers in terms of childbirth support and breastfeeding.

We can create new positions in hospitals to assist doctors and midwives with the emotional support mothers and parents need.

- **Mothers: Provide knowledge to mothers.**

We must communicate on the way to give birth and the options mothers have to go with the natural phases of labour and childbirth. Mothers can learn how to connect with themselves, understand the process, learn how the woman's body operates during labour and gain confidence in their own capabilities. We only need to know a few notions of our pelvis and perineum to understand how to embody our body. We must also fully integrate that we are giving birth no one else.

Our whole being is in control in a focused way while we are surrendering to the experience. Our body knows, mothers can learn to become active and accompany the process of childbirth. Doctors and midwifes don't give birth for us, they are here to assist, guide us and take over if needed.

The training we receive in childbirth preparation classes is vague, boring, and difficult to apply when you finally are in the heat of the moment of childbirth. It can be much more specific, playful and easily assimilated by the mind and body.

Centuries ago, mothers and children used to commonly die at birth, nowadays we have gone too far with the medical assistance. It's as if most of us go the hospital and say, "OK, get it out of there, I don't want to know how and I don't want to feel anything." Or other mothers, like me, who were terrified by the idea of a baby coming out of their vagina. Not knowing how far the pain can go in intensity during labour is extremely scary.

And on top of that, hospitals put mothers through sanitised, restrictive procedures and protocols. Most of these procedures do not hold solid grounds anymore.

When mothers give birth fully aware and connected to their body and baby, the medical teams gain priceless time with less over assisted mothers and medical procedures. Perhaps doctors and midwives would have a bit more time to accompany the mother and give her the space to feel the powerful and magical moments. Rather than reacting with stress and paying the consequences later at home personally.

I've heard it on both sides, mothers frightened, out of control, missing the moment, reacting, not responding to the situation. And the medical staff in a reacting mode, complaining about the lack of time and implication, the exhaustion, and the frustration they feel when they get home after a very long, extended shift.

More and more mothers create a birth list with their wishes of how they want to give birth. While this is a very good initiative, it is hard for the hospitals to follow. There is not enough staff nor means to assure a personalised experience to each mother. And when things don't go the way the mother would like them to, it only creates more frustration and disappointment. We can't expect all the efforts to be made on one side. However, if women learn and efficiently prepare for birth, a birth list can be a very good ally and would be easier to include in the hospitals' protocols.

As Bob Proctor said: "You have to understand something about your computer if you're going to work with it." Well, it's the same with birth, you have to understand something about your body and powers within you to work with it.

If you are frustrated with what hospitals or society impose on you as a future mother, you've got to learn about yourself.

For my first successful pregnancy, I had no idea how to give birth and I was terrified. It's not the few theory classes at the hospital that helped me understand my body and how to manage the pain. You have to prepare your body with specific physiological exercises, with repetition, to fully embody it.

Just like a marathon, you must prepare for birth. The knowledge will be metabolised spontaneously, and it will give you that trust in yourself. And with selfcare and meditation, you will be able to work with your body and mind in a more confident and grounded way.

### o   Oneness VS Self-centredness and Dependence

So, we have seen how to take care of ourselves and how to learn to love ourselves. It's a matter of comprehending how to use our higher faculties and dimmer the ego. Loving ourselves not in a self-conscious way but in a way to find love within ourselves and nurture that light we all have in us, and that allows us to love others.

What I love is that today we can openly talk about energy, higher vibration, power of the self, love, oneness without being a spiritual person. I am a spiritual person but what I mean is that it is accessible to all. Today, many professors, doctors and neuroscientists talk about all this and how it exists even though we can't see nor touch it.

Daniel J. Siegel, M.D. is a clinical professor of Psychiatry at the UCLA School of Medicine and the founding co-director of the Mindful Awareness Research Centre at UCLA. He explains in his latest book *Intraconnected, (Me + We)*, that our perception of the world is through our personal lens with our beliefs. The world through our lens is very small and it keeps us separate and alone.

What if we don't need lenses, what if we remove them and discover how large and beautiful our world really is. We can learn to shift our perception of who we are, that we are not that separate 'me' self, but that we are all 'one'. I am, is all of us. We are all one source of energy, we are all connected, we are all this love.

Self-love doesn't mean isolating ourselves; this would be living in separateness. Self-love is nurturing ourselves first, then sharing with others. Like the neuroscientist Richard Davidson says in the *Dalai Lama's guide to happiness:* "We are social animals." We need to live together and we need to share. Life would be meaningless if we were alone and didn't care for anyone.

The Dalai Lama repeats again and again: "We are seven to eight billion human beings, we are the same. We have to think, we are all human brothers and sisters. We have to live on this planet together. I firmly believe, we really need to concert oneness of seven to eight billion human beings." This may sound very simple and unrealistic, but it's the only way and it can be done.

I have seen people who when they take the path of self-development and the search to inner happiness, become quite selfish and consequently isolate themselves, to end-up feeling lonelier. Authenticity of the self can be found with true self-care, with true introspection which then allows to share and care for others. When we take the path of self-development and inner healing we do it for our happiness first but also to share it around us and inspire others to do the same.

**The tricky notions to remember here are self-love doesn't mean self-centredness and separateness. And oneness doesn't mean depending on others.**

When you feel anxious about the idea of giving birth, things going wrong, not being the right mother to your newborn, not knowing if your way of doing is right or wrong; the answers are within you. Look within for the soothing comfort. Advice from outside sources is here to help you and guide you but the trust and love will come from within.

We must stop desperately looking for approval from others, outward comfort, outward recognition; this is dependence. The material world and exterior sources will never make you deeply happy. The power is not from outside the self, you can spend a lifetime running after something you had in you all along. I can say this because gosh it took me twenty years to finally understand this and dig in there.

That love, trust, confidence, compassion and warm kindness is in you. You can stop looking for it in things or people. Once you tap in there, you can connect with the oneness we are all part of and start showing up differently in the world.

Again, Richard Davidson explains it so well in *Dalai Lama's guide to happiness*. "Authentic happiness is not dependent on external circumstances. External rewards will never be enough. LOVE is our evolutionary capacity to cooperate, communicate and connect, this allowed our species to thrive."

**The power of the self is our soul, the light, the energy we all are, and we all come from. The Dalai Lama calls it our Buddha nature; Deepak Chopra calls it the unified field; Napoleon Hill the infinite intelligence; Bob Proctor the natural laws of the Universe or God; Rebecca Campbell, source or universal energy.**

Now there is no magic, it's not by looking out the window at the sky hoping something will change that the deep self-referral will reveal itself to you. Even though connecting to nature and the elements will ground you in the present. Being in the present is getting a glimpse of this universal source. The self-referral can be truly felt by practicing meditation primarily, taking that time of stillness for you to feel. Then implementing in your daily life the other tools that speak to your heart and make you feel good.

This with repetition will change your paradigm, your mechanical habits that were leading you nowhere. It will allow you to get in touch with your soul, with your true essence, with the universal energy, with your Buddha nature.

Our world is already changing, we can see it on social media, we can see it in marketing, in publicity, in the industries. Each of us have a role in our field; it's a matter of all being more aware and participating to the change the world needs. If we all do something, little by little, we will build solid foundations for a new way of living in harmony with the earth and interacting with one another.

o   **How Do We Give Our Children the Right Seeds?**

With all the notions in this book, you are creating intention and intention is extremely powerful, it's like a laser. Intention is where you want to go, it's very precise and it's how you want to go there. How do you want your children to live and what qualities would you like them to embody? As mothers, we have a huge role to play in how we want the world to evolve and how our children will live in it.

This is not a 'have to', 'must do', 'be the perfect mum' thing. It's about YOU, nurturing yourself and choosing the tools and methods that work for you. Awakening your consciousness to a different way of living and vibrating.

By acquiring the knowledge in this book, by developing your awareness and by taking care of yourself, you are naturally preparing and providing a happy and balanced environment for your child. By implementing the tools for the body and mind with repetition, thus changing your paradigm and your habits, you will breathe, move and vibrate more in harmony with who you are and with loving kindness towards yourself.

The magic about this is that the outcome for each of you will be different because you are unique. Just like our DNA is different for each one of us, the results in your well-being and life will be different; they will be yours, that's the beauty.

Talking about DNA, it's also about how you were brought into the world and how your baby will be born into the world. When you experience childbirth with the tools, with the trust and the connection with yourself and your baby, you are creating your environment. You are choosing what serves you, what you are taking with you and what you are leaving behind.

You are surrendering to the experience of childbirth and motherhood, you are showing the way to your child. Your baby is being welcomed into the world in an authentic and true way, your way.

By adopting some or all these loving and nurturing tools for yourself, you are creating an invisible and powerful harmony or flow that your child is directly bathed in. It's like the natural forces of the Universe at action; there is an infinite organising power in it as described by Deepak Chopra, it's "the movements of galaxies, the movements of stars, (…) the cycles of the seasons, the biological rhythms of our bodies," it operates by nature, instinctively.

As we discussed earlier what a paradigm is, Bob Proctor also explains how the baby's paradigm is formed. "The baby has been inundated with trivia, the conversations that are going on around the baby, things that are deemed to be important, worrying about this, worrying about that (…) All of this trivia ultimately enslaves the baby. It becomes part of the baby's paradigm."

Yes, this is life, but you are learning how to handle the daily trivia, to not get trapped in it and to have the insight. You are learning to live with presence in the present. The noise and stress won't affect your baby because he or she already profoundly knows his or her mother is in tune and is working with the power of the self.

By changing your habits and living more in tune with yourself, giving yourself love and understanding, giving yourself time, knowing you have the tools, that you are not alone, you are naturally transmitting these powers in a grounded energy to your baby.

If we set the right environment by working the 'self' with unconditional love before birth, by creating your childbirth environment wherever you are, and nurturing this during the first year of childhood, a promising paradigm will be formed for your child. Your child after being immerged in this not perfect but compassionate harmony will simply develop the qualities of love, compassion, altruism, and faith.

These are the values our world urgently needs. This is how we can change things, with love, with the natural attributes our children will embody.

The most 'ah ah' moment for me while writing this book was when I heard that science had recently proved this. I had almost finished writing my book, when Dan Harris and Richard Davidson released the five-part series of the *Dalai Lama's guide to happiness,* I have mentioned several times in the book.

The neuroscientist Richard Davidson explains, and I will allow myself quite a long quote: "Certain kinds of meditation practices including compassion practices can alter our epigenetics and this can be passed down at least a few generations. Science of epigenetics is the science of how our genes are regulated. Research has clearly shown that by cultivating compassion in this lifetime, it can actually benefit on our future generations. This, in a real biological mechanistic way."

"Current research on pregnant woman, who learnt to practice compassion and meditation, show that it is beneficial for the women but also for their babies. When the babies are born, researchers get a sample of blood from the umbilical cord and through that can get an epigenetic snapshot of the foetus and actually see the impact of the mother practicing compassion on the epigenetics of the foetus."

How amazing is this? Science just back-up my experiential and recent intuitive knowledge!

First of all, if you apply these principles, your child will have a solid and balanced paradigm. When your child's ego talks or paradigm of fear shows up, she/he will know how to handle it and won't feel alone and powerless in our divided world; despite the constant feed of information and external noise. Secondly, I believe that by awakening one after the other, it won't be a divided world anymore but a world of community and unity.

Just as Mahatma Gandhi says: "Let us work together for unity and love." Or "Our ability to reach unity in diversity will be the beauty and the test of our civilisation."

The world is awakening, and our role as loving, divine mothers is to set the right preamble to the future on earth. Each one of us can participate as it matters for you, for your child and for the collective.

I listened to a beautiful podcast from Tara Brach in conversation with Mingyur Rinpoche, a Tibetan Buddhist and meditation master. The talk was fascinating and finished with a notion that spoke to my heart. They talked about the fact that often we feel discouraged as a person in our actions when there is a global crisis. We feel it as one person in front of one big problem.

We feel helpless and small. But the truth is that the entire world depends on the individual, on each person, on you and on me. The collective starts by the individual and the big problem isn't such a big problem anymore.

In motherhood, we can reach a more respectful, natural and authentic way of connecting with ourselves, with our baby and the world around us. And it starts with you and me.